Lead from the Edge

A Quiet Rebellion Against the Life You Outgrew

Andrea Ubhi

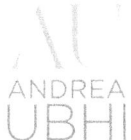

Lead from the Edge © 2025 Andrea Ubhi

All rights reserved.

No part of this publication may be reproduced, distributed, or transmitted in any form or by any means, including photocopying, recording, or other electronic or mechanical methods, without the prior written permission of the author, except in the case of brief quotations embodied in reviews or critical articles.

This book is a work of nonfiction. The names and identifying details of some individuals have been changed to protect their privacy. The views expressed are those of the author based on personal experience and reflection.

For permissions, rights, or bulk purchases, please contact:

andreaubhi.com

Published by Andrea Ubhi Ltd.

ISBN: 978-1-9162400-1-8

First Edition 2025

All proceeds from this book are donated to Asha Nepal, a grassroots charity supporting women and children survivors of trafficking.

For those standing quietly on the edge.
This is for you.

Introduction

The Edge Is Where Everything Changed

There's a moment — and if you're reading this, you've likely had your own — when the life that once fit... no longer does.

You've done the things. Worn the titles. Tick-boxed the success.

And yet — something inside is restless. Not broken. Just *done* with the performance.

This book was born at the edge of that moment.

After illness, burnout, and a life that once looked great on paper, I found myself somewhere I didn't expect: questioning everything.

My pace. My ambition. My identity. My definition of strength. And what surprised me most was this:

The edge didn't break me.

It clarified me.

Introduction

This Book Is for You If…

You're the one who's always been capable.

Held it all. Done it all. You don't crumble — you carry. But you're tired. Not in the way sleep can fix — in the way *reality* needs to change.

This is for you if you're in transition, or reinvention, or recovery. If you're over performing. If you're craving something slower, deeper, truer. If you're ready to stop proving and start becoming.

This Is Not a Blueprint. It's a Compass.

I'm not here to give you a five-step formula. I know you don't need one.

What you'll find in these pages are stories, metaphors, and moments — truths discovered in business meetings, during chemo, in silences, on summits, and in the kitchen.

You'll find reflections.
You'll find calm.
You'll find permission:
To stop climbing someone else's mountain.
To stop chasing a version of success that was never your dream.
To come home — to the self beneath the performance.

What to Expect Inside

Each chapter explores a different edge:
Of strength. Of truth. Of self.

And at the end of every chapter, you'll find practical reflection prompts, micro-actions, and short stories — to help you not just read, but integrate.

Some chapters will feel like deep breaths.

Introduction

Others might challenge you.

All of them are invitations to lead differently — starting from within.

This Is Where It Starts

This isn't a leadership book in the traditional sense.

But it *is* a book about leadership — the kind that begins at the edges of who you used to be, and dares to become something truer.

You don't have to shout to lead.

You don't have to climb to prove.

You don't have to break down to begin again.

You just have to be willing... to stand at the edge, and listen.

Let's begin.

Andrea

Part One
Arriving at the Edge

Chapter 1
The Edge is Real

"*Sometimes the bravest and most important thing you can do is just show up.*"
— *Brené Brown*

When Success Didn't Feel Like Success

There's a strange moment that happens when you hit a milestone — and it doesn't sit well in your heart. You get the award. The title. The numbers. The recognition.

And instead of feeling fulfilled... you feel hollow. Tired. Disconnected. Or nothing at all.

Success — on paper — doesn't always feel like success in your body.

From the outside, it looked like everything was working. And in a way, it was.

But inside?

I was running on fumes. I was pushing through instead of showing up. And I didn't feel successful — I felt scattered.

This was one of the turning points.

Not a breakdown. But a quiet *realisation*: I had built something that looked incredible — but didn't feel like *me* anymore. This chapter is about that shift. From chasing success to choosing alignment. From performance to presence. From loud wins to *real* ones.

The Performance of Success

Success can become a costume.

The business that looks shiny on the outside. The calendar full of important meetings. The LinkedIn-worthy milestones. The well-practiced smile. The curated life.

We chase what we were taught to chase. Titles. Growth. Praise. And when we get there, we're surprised to find it doesn't always feel the way we hoped. Because a life that's impressive but misaligned - still leaves you tired, still leaves you lonely, still leaves you wondering why it's not enough.

And here's what makes it tricky:

You can be deeply grateful... and still quietly unhappy.

You can be successful... and still feel lost.

You can be proud... and still feel *not quite right*.

That doesn't make you unthankful. It makes you aware. This is the moment when performance starts to peel away —and the truth starts to breathe again.

The Invisible Cost of Looking Successful

Looking successful is a full-time job. And sometimes, it's one you never applied for — it just came with the territory. The cost isn't just energy. It's *identity*.

You become the polished version of yourself — the one who's

got it sorted. The one who smiles, responds, delivers, inspires. The one who doesn't fall apart. Ever.

And that version? She might be stunning on the outside...but she's often held together by adrenaline, pressure, and the unspoken fear of *"what if I stop?"*

There was a time, when my children were small, that the exhaustion was almost cellular. I'd survive the night in broken fragments — two hours here, forty-five minutes there — and then morning would arrive like a test I hadn't revised for. Again.

I remember plastering on a smile. Wiping faces. Packing bags. Trying to be functional when what I really needed was to lie down in a dark room and sleep.

But that wasn't the script. So I dug deep.

Really deep.

The kind of deep where you forget what it feels like to *not* be coping. The kind of deep where you're running on reserves you didn't even know you had. Like scraping the last teaspoon of honey from the jar — even after it is all gone.

It may have looked like strength, but my body remembers it differently. It remembers the tension in my jaw. The fatigue behind my eyes. The pressure in my chest with every "I'm fine" I said that wasn't quite true.

We're told that keeping up appearances is noble. But sometimes, it's just suppression in good lighting.

If I could go back and whisper something to that younger version of me? I'd say: *Don't dig so deep. Earn less. Spend less. And spend more energy on yourself — your rest, your joy, your soul.* Because you were never meant to be a bottomless well. Even the strongest woman deserves to stop... and refill.

The exhaustion is cumulative.

Not just physical — *emotional.*

You become hyper-aware of how others see you.

You carry the weight of every "I'm so inspired by you" like it's a fragile glass you're not allowed to drop. But here's what I know now:

There's a version of success that doesn't drain you.

There's a way of leading that doesn't cost your well-being.

There's a way back to *you* — but it starts with stepping out of the role.

Redefining What Matters Now

At some point, you stop asking, *"What do I want to achieve?"*

And you start asking, *"What do I want to feel?"*

Success begins to look less like a podium... and more like a peaceful morning. Less like applause... and more like presence. Less like *"What did I do today?"*

And more like *"Who was I while I did it?"*

You don't have to want less. You just want different.

You want:

- Energy that lasts beyond the win
- Work that feeds your soul — not your CV
- A schedule that allows space to think, move, breathe
- Connections that feel nourishing, not performative
- Joy, not just accomplishment
- Impact that doesn't cost your health

Success doesn't have to be dramatic. It just has to be *real*. The world might still reward the loud, the fast, the visible. But your life? It rewards the true.

And what matters now is not how high you climb —but how *you* feel on the way up.

Your Values Are the New Metrics

I used to measure success by speed. By volume. By how many things were ticked off, how much praise arrived, how productive I was.

But when everything changed — my body, my energy, my life — the old metrics stopped making sense.

Now?

Success looks different. It's not the pace — it's the *fit*. Not how much you do — but how aligned you feel while doing it.

You start to measure:

- How light your body feels at the end of the day
- Whether your schedule reflects your priorities
- How calm your mind is when you lie down to sleep
- How often you laugh (really laugh)
- How many decisions you make that honour your boundaries, not just your role
- How much of what you do is driven by joy — not just duty

A few years ago, I worked with a life coach who helped me explore my core values — not the ones I thought I *should* have, but the ones that actually shaped how I felt when life felt good. Back then, my top three values were completely different from what they are now. Several years on, I've changed.

Now, my values are: **Joy. Calm. Adventure.**

These aren't aspirational. They're *foundational*. They're how I know I'm living well — even if the decision I'm making doesn't look "right" on paper. Even if it doesn't maximise profit or approval.

When a decision feels deeply right in my soul — but not conventionally wise from a business perspective — I remind myself: This is my joy. My calm. My adventure.

And that is my success.

And when I make choices that don't align with those values — even if they're "strategically smart" — they feel off. They feel wrong. Eventually, my body tells me. My energy dips. I disconnect. Until I stop, and remember: *I'm off-track. Not with the world — with myself.*

How to Find Your Core Values

1. Remember a moment when you felt most alive, peaceful, or proud of yourself. What values were present in that moment? Freedom? Creativity? Connection?
2. Write down 10–15 words that matter to you. Then circle the top 5. Then 3. Don't overthink. Notice what feels like a *yes* in your body.
3. Ask yourself: "When I feel aligned, which values are being honoured?" "When I feel drained, which values have I been ignoring?"

Try them on. Like favourite clothes. Use them to guide small decisions first — then bigger ones.

Because your values aren't just a list. They're a compass. And when you follow them — *really* follow them — your version of success might look different from the world's... but it will *feel* exactly right to you.

. . .

When your values become your metrics, everything shifts. You stop asking, *"Am I doing enough?"* And start asking, *"Am I doing what matters — to me?"* That's when the pressure starts to loosen. And the real success begins to unfold.

The Inner Compass, Not the External Map

For most of our lives, we were handed a map.

It came with clear instructions:

- Climb this ladder
- Hit these milestones
- Achieve this level of income, visibility, admiration

If we followed the map, we were told, we'd end up somewhere good. And maybe we did. But somewhere along the way… we looked around and thought,

"This isn't quite it."

That's when the map stops working. Because it was never ours to begin with. Now? We're following something different: A *compass*.

It doesn't give detailed directions. It doesn't tell what our lives *should* look like. It simply points in the direction of what feels true. Toward peace. Toward presence. Toward energy that expands, not depletes.

You don't always know what's around the bend. But you can feel when you're walking toward the right thing — even if no one else gets it.

The compass doesn't promise efficiency. It promises *integrity*. And when you start following it? That's when life stops being a performance — and starts becoming a path that actually feels like yours.

Reflection — What Does Success Mean to You Now?

- Pause for a moment.
- Step off the treadmill.
- Breathe.

We're taught what success looks like long before we get to ask what it *feels* like.

The grades. The house. The title. The applause.

But the problem with success built for someone else's life…is that even when you reach it, it doesn't feel like ours. This is our chance to revisit the definition.

To ask — not what looks good on paper, but what sits right in our soul.

Journal Moment

- What did success used to mean for you —and who handed you that definition?
- What version of success have you outgrown, but still feel pressure to perform?
- What does success feel like in your body — lightness, ease, alignment, peace?
- If you weren't trying to prove anything to anyone… what would you do differently this week?
- What if success wasn't something to chase — but something to come home to?

You don't have to burn it all down. But you're allowed to stop chasing a version of life that doesn't fit anymore.

Pause. Reflect. Realign.

This is your permission to leave the borrowed path.
  To stop performing for a definition you didn't choose.
  Success doesn't need to be louder — it just needs to be *yours*.

Edge Move — Redefine It Out Loud

This week, write your own definition of success. Make it honest. Quiet. Messy, even.
  It might sound like:

- "Success is waking up with peace in my chest."
- "Success is saying no without guilt."
- "Success is doing meaningful work with time left to hike."
- "Success is how I treat myself when no one's watching."
- "Success is freedom — to be, to rest, to create, to live."

  Then: **Say it out loud.**
  To yourself. To someone else. Maybe even online — if it feels bold.
  Because the more you live your version of success… the less the old one will pull you back.

Chapter 2
The Edge of Joy

"Life is tough, my darling, but so are you."
— *Stephanie Bennett-Henry*

Joy Isn't a Luxury — It's a Sign of Healing

We're taught that joy comes *after* the work. After the crisis. After the achievement. After the schedule is clear and the inbox is empty and the house is clean and the responsibilities are handled. But that version of joy? It rarely arrives. Because the finish line keeps moving.

Here's another truth:
Joy isn't what comes after healing.
Joy is what signals that healing has begun.

When we've lived in survival mode, joy can feel optional. Silly. Even selfish.

But it's not.

Joy is your body telling you: *"There is space now."* There's breath again. There's presence. There's enough steadiness that you can feel something more than just tension. It doesn't have to be loud or performative. It can be a spark. A second of soft. The quiet moment where you notice beauty — and don't rush past it. Like the first wildflowers after winter. Not required. Not functional. But full of meaning.

Joy doesn't ask you to be fixed. It asks you to be open.

Not to force it — but to *let it in.*

Why Joy Can Feel Unfamiliar After Pain

After you've walked through pain, joy can feel… suspicious.

Too light. Too bright. Too much. You might flinch at it. Hold your breath around it. Worry it won't last — or that you don't deserve it.

That's not a character flaw. It's what happens when your system has been trained to expect the next blow. After grief, joy feels fragile. After burnout, it feels indulgent. After survival, it can even feel unsafe. When you've spent months — or years — living in high alert, joy doesn't always feel welcome. It feels unfamiliar. Foreign. Maybe even a little… dangerous.

This is a nervous system trying to protect you. Not because it doesn't want joy — but because it's learned to scan for threat. So if joy feels uncomfortable — it's not because it's wrong. It's because your body forgot what safety feels like.

But you can remind it. Gently. Gradually. Kindly. Joy isn't just something to feel.

It's something to *relearn*.

We're Wired to Prepare for the Worst, Not Feel the Best

Our nervous system isn't designed to prioritise happiness. It's designed to keep us alive. Which means it's always scanning for what might go wrong — not what's already going right.

This is ancient wiring.

Your brain's first question isn't *"What feels good?"* It's *"What might hurt me?"* That's why we rehearse worst-case scenarios. That's why we feel more in control when we're anticipating disaster than when we're resting in joy.

Joy requires vulnerability. Presence. The willingness to stop bracing for the next blow — and feel something good now. And that's not always easy. If our body tenses when something good happens — that's not a failure of mindset. It's a sign we've been living in protection mode for too long.

But here's the hope: You can teach your system that it's safe to soften. Safe to enjoy. Safe to let good things in — without rushing to earn them, justify them, or prepare to lose them.

Joy doesn't mean danger. It means we're finally stepping out of survival.

Small Joy as a Way Back to Wholeness

You don't need to overhaul your life to feel joy again. You just need one opening. Not a grand gesture. Not a perfect day. Just a small, honest *yes* to something that makes your shoulders drop.

Because wholeness doesn't return all at once. It comes back in tiny ways — usually unannounced.

It looks like:

- Laughing unexpectedly at something silly
- Finding a moment of stillness in a noisy day
- Letting the sun warm your face and noticing how good it feels
- Breathing fully without rushing to the next thing

These aren't distractions. They're repairs. These are the micro-signals that say, *"I'm still here. I still know how to feel."* You don't have to force it. You don't have to be "ready." You just have to let it happen — even briefly. Because the path back to yourself often begins with a smile you didn't see coming.

During recovery from Non-Hodgkins lymphoma, there was a moment — just an ordinary day — when I realised I wasn't tired. Not energised. Not buzzing. Just... *not tired*. I hadn't felt that in months. Maybe years. And in that moment, it felt like joy. Not the jump-up-and-down kind. The kind that settles softly in your chest and whispers, *"You're coming back."*

Joy Doesn't Need a Reason — Just a Little Space

We're so used to earning everything. Rest must be earned.

Success must be proven. And joy? We tuck it behind achievement, survival, or someone else's permission slip. But joy doesn't work like that. It doesn't arrive on a schedule or wait for things to be neat. Joy doesn't need a reason. It just needs *space*.

It's easy to think:

- *"I can enjoy this after the launch."*
- *"Once I fix this, then I'll let myself relax."*
- *"It would be silly to enjoy anything right now — not when things are still messy."*

But some of the most honest joy comes *in the middle* of the mess. The moment you pause in a day that isn't going well — and sip your coffee slowly. The laugh that bubbles up in a hospital corridor. The song you dance to in a kitchen full of laundry and unanswered emails.

That joy? That's not irresponsibility. That's resilience. You don't have to explain it. You don't have to tone it down. You just have to *let it exist* — even briefly. It belongs. Even here.

Especially here.

The First Wildflowers After the Fire

After a wildfire, the ground doesn't stay bare. Before the trees return, before the forest reshapes itself — something unexpected happens.

The first thing to grow? Wildflowers. Bright. Fragile. Unapologetically alive. They emerge through the ash and charred soil, softening the destruction.

Not because the land is healed. But because it's *healing*.

That's what joy is. The wildflowers after your fire. It's your body and spirit's first brave act of return. Not because everything's perfect — but because something inside you knows: *life goes on*.

Joy is proof that softness survives. That beauty insists on blooming — even when the timeline makes no sense. You don't need to rebuild everything before you let colour back in. You just need to allow something tender to take root.

Joy doesn't wait for permission.

Reflection — Let Joy Feel Safe Again

Let yourself reflect — slowly, honestly, gently. This isn't about chasing happiness. It's about allowing joy to return — without the fear that it will vanish again.

Because when life has been hard, unpredictable, or heavy, joy can feel... dangerous. Like it might slip through your fingers. Like it's too tender to trust. Like you haven't earned it yet.

But joy isn't something to prove yourself worthy of. It's something that remembers who you are — even when you forget.

Journal Moment

- What kind of joy feels safe to you right now — playful, quiet, steady, private?
- Where have you been holding back from joy, believing you need to "deserve" it first?
- What kind of joy have you been waiting for — that you might actually be allowed to choose today?
- What's one small, quiet joy you can return to this week — just for you, no audience, no performance?
- What would it look like to trust that joy isn't fragile — that it can hold you, even here?

This isn't about bold declarations of happiness.
    It's about letting joy take up space again.
    In your morning breath.
    In your slow coffee.
    In the way sunlight lands on your arm.

Pause. Reflect. Realign.

Joy doesn't require a permission slip.
    It's not a reward — it's a reminder.
    That you are still here.
    And life still wants to meet you with softness.

Edge Move — Let Joy In

This week, let one small joy land.
    Not because you earned it. Not because it makes sense.
    Just because you can.

Lead from the Edge

- Say yes to something light.
- Move slowly through something beautiful.
- Let yourself laugh before you explain why you're allowed to.
- Sit in a pocket of sunshine.
- Listen to the song again — the one that makes your chest ache (in the good way).
- And don't rush it.

This is joy. Not after the storm.
Inside it.

Chapter 3
Your Voice, Your Pace

"*If you want to fly, you have to give up everything that weighs you down.*"
Toni Morrison

When You Realise You've Been Performing

There comes a moment — quiet, almost imperceptible — when we realise we've been performing. Not on a stage.

Just... in life.

We've been moving fast, speaking confidently, responding quickly, smiling often — even when something inside us was asking for a different rhythm. It's not fake. It's just survival.

We adapt to what's expected. We meet the tone of the room. We keep up — until one day, we wonder... *"Why am I trying so hard to keep up at all?"*

This is not a failure. It's a noticing.

It's the beginning of return. To our own tone. Our own timing. Our own voice — the one that doesn't rush, perform, or over-explain.

The world didn't ask for that version. But our body, our spirit, our peace... did.

And now, we're ready to listen.

The Pressure to Be "On"

We learn early that the world responds best when we're switched on.

Bright. Quick. Engaged. Capable. Smiling.

We keep the pace. We finish the sentence. We hold the room. We never drop the ball. And we're praised for it — even applauded. But beneath the performance is a quiet pressure:

- To always be articulate
- To respond immediately
- To match the tempo of a room we never agreed to
- To stay composed, even when something inside us is quietly fraying

Being "on" becomes a reflex. We lose touch with our true rhythm — because we're so used to matching everyone else's. We answer before we've even thought. We say yes, not because it's right — but because silence feels awkward. We move fast, not because we're in a hurry — but because we've always been expected to be the one who moves fast.

It's automatic.
Conditioned.
Efficient, even.
But it's not you.

Somewhere in there, your actual pace — your truth, your timing — got overridden by performance. By pleasing. By the muscle memory of being the capable one.

What if you paused next time?

What if you didn't fill the silence?

What if you let the question be asked — and answered with your body, not your habit?

That's where your voice lives. Not in the automatic yes — but in the *considered no*. The grounded *maybe*.

The brave pause.

And at some point, the mask gets heavy. The applause starts to feel hollow. And your nervous system starts asking: *"Can we breathe now?"* You weren't meant to live on high alert. You weren't meant to prove your presence every time you enter a room.

You're allowed to rest your voice. You're allowed to find your natural tempo again — even if it confuses people at first. They'll adjust.

And more importantly — so will you.

Fast Isn't Always Strong — It's Just Fast

We glorify speed. Quick answers. Rapid growth. Instant replies. Fast becomes shorthand for smart, capable, driven. But fast isn't always strong.

Sometimes fast is just... *habit*. A nervous system on autopilot. A fear of being caught behind. A subtle belief that if we slow down, we'll lose ground — or worse, be forgotten.

But real strength?

It's not in the pace. It's in the *presence*. It takes strength to pause before answering. To take a breath before reacting. To listen fully instead of filling the silence. To admit, "I don't know yet," and not feel rushed to find a perfect sentence.

Strong is not the person sprinting through every hour. Strong is the person who knows their own rhythm — and doesn't abandon it just to keep up.

Fast can be helpful. But it's not holy.

The real power is in knowing when to go fast... and when to *stand still*.

Your Pace Is Allowed to Change

There's no gold star for keeping the same pace forever. Who you were five years ago may have thrived on urgency. Deadlines. Back-to-back meetings. Energy that never stopped buzzing.

But maybe now...

- You want slower mornings.
- You need more space between things.
- You answer more gently.
- You move with more intention — and less adrenaline.

That's not losing your edge. That's *finding your alignment*. Pace is seasonal. You're allowed to move differently now — even if the world doesn't understand.

You don't owe anyone the same version of yourself forever.

After chemo, my brain slowed down.

It felt like whole pockets of cells had been blasted and gone. If you asked me a question, I'd need a moment to find the answer. Sometimes I'd pause mid-sentence, just trying to remember the end of my own train of thought.

It was frustrating. Humbling. But somewhere in that slowness, I found something valuable:

The *pause*.

I used to speak quickly — instinctively. Say the first thing, then course-correct. Talk my way through uncertainty.

Now, I pause.

Not because I'm unsure — but because I'm finally sure. Sure that I want to speak *from* truth, not toward it. Sure that silence doesn't need to be filled. Sure that slower often means stronger.

My brain cells may have renewed, but I've kept the lesson:

Pause before replying.

Let the words catch up with the truth. Sometimes the hardest part isn't slowing down — it's letting go of the person who needed to move so fast. You don't have to explain the shift. You just have to honour it. Because the goal isn't to keep up.

It's to stay true.

Your Voice Doesn't Have to Be Loud to Be Heard

We've been taught that to be taken seriously, we need to turn the volume up. Be bolder. Be clearer. Speak faster. Speak more. Raise our hand, our voice, our energy — or risk being overlooked. But volume isn't the only way to lead.

Presence is.

There's power in a calm voice that doesn't waver. In a thoughtful pause that holds the room. In saying only what needs to be said — and letting it land. Our power doesn't depend on projection.

It depends on *alignment*.

Some voices carry because they're loud. Yours can carry because it's clear. Rooted. Unapologetic — even if it's quiet. You don't have to shout to be heard. You just have to speak from truth — not performance. And when you do, you stop speaking for approval… and start speaking for impact.

The Tide, Not the Clock

Clocks measure time in sharp lines. Minutes. Deadlines. Alarms.

Tides measure time in rhythm. In rise and return. In pause and pull. In knowing that every surge is followed by stillness — and stillness is not failure.

We are not a clock. We are a tide.

We don't have to match the urgency of someone else's pace. We're allowed to move differently — more slowly, more intuitively — led by something quieter, deeper, and older than urgency.

Imagine if we judged the sea for not rushing. For retreating. For pausing. For shifting in its own time. And yet — we don't. We trust it. We know the ocean is still powerful… even when it's still.

Clocks belong to productivity. Tides belong to nature.

In the same way, you're allowed to reset your timing. To slow. To rise. To pull back. To arrive.

Power isn't measured by how fast you speak, reply, launch, or act. It's felt in your *gravity*. The presence you carry. The rhythm you honour. The truth you move in. Let the others watch the clock. You listen to the tide.

Reflection — What Pace Is Actually Yours?

Let yourself check in. Not with the world's speed — but with your own. You've spent so long matching other people's rhythms, you might've forgotten you get to choose your own.

Pace is personal. And too often, we confuse busyness with purpose. Energy with aliveness. Momentum with meaning.

But what if the real power is in slowing down?

In listening for your natural tempo — not the one you were trained into, but the one that allows your nervous system, your creativity, and your truth to breathe.

Journal Moment

- Where have you been rushing — not because it's urgent, but because it's familiar?
- What part of your day (or life) still feels like it's trying to "keep up"?
- If no one were watching, what pace would feel most true — not just today, but this season of life?
- What would it sound like to speak in your own voice again — not louder, just clearer?
- Where could you slow down — not as an act of laziness, but as a return to alignment?

You don't have to be more energetic. More polished. More efficient. More anything.

You just have to be more *you* — at the volume, rhythm, and speed that honours where you are now.

Pause. Reflect. Realign.

You're not falling behind. You're falling back into your natural pace. And from that place — clarity comes.

Creativity comes. Peace returns.

Edge Move — Choose Your Rhythm

This week, choose one rhythm — and celebrate it.

- Speak slower than usual
- Walk at your natural pace, not someone else's stride
- Let yourself pause before replying

- Say, "I'll come back to you on that," instead of rushing to answer
- Take five more minutes. Say fewer words. Rest in the silence between them.

Let the world meet *your* tempo. You don't need to race to keep your place. You're already here.

Chapter 4
Living Fully, Not Loudly

"Our deepest wishes are whispers of our authentic self. We must learn to respect them. We must learn to listen."

— *Sarah Ban Breathnach*

When Loud Was the Goal

There was a time when louder felt like the way forward. Bigger presence. Bigger energy. Bigger visibility. Post more. Say more. Be more. The world rewards the extroverted, the available, the always-on.

So we learn to turn ourselves up. We believe that to be successful — to be *seen* — we must be louder. Clearer. Bolder. Brighter. All the time.

It's not that loud is wrong. But when loud becomes the *only* measure of aliveness… we lose something quieter, but far more essential.

Loudness can become a mask for uncertainty. A placeholder

for presence. A substitute for meaning. Eventually, something inside you whispers:

"*What if I don't want to shout anymore?*"

And that whisper? That's the beginning of something real.

The Exhaustion of Being "On" All the Time

Being "on" isn't just a state — it's a performance. You smile even when you're tired. You post when you'd rather pause. You say yes out of habit, because saying no feels like losing relevance.

There's always one more thing to keep up with:

- A message to respond to
- A caption to write
- A platform to update
- A presence to maintain

And slowly, the line between *you* and your performance begins to blur. You feel it in your body — that quiet resistance. The sigh before you open the app. The weight in your chest when you know you need to show up, but your soul's already left the room.

There is a cost to constant visibility. And it's often paid in clarity, rest, and depth.

But here's the gift:

You can step off the stage. Even if no one notices — especially if no one notices. You're not here to impress strangers.

You're here to live.

And sometimes, the most powerful thing you can do...is *disappear on purpose*, and return to yourself.

People say you have to love yourself first.

I used to roll my eyes at that — it felt vague and self-indulgent. Surely it's better to be loving, helpful, outward-facing?

But the truth is: if you're on empty, you don't have anything to give. You can't pour from a dry cup. You can't lead well when you're breathless. You can't support others if you've abandoned yourself in the process.

It's like the oxygen masks on a plane. They always say: put yours on first. Not because you're selfish — but because if you pass out from lack of oxygen, you can't help *anyone* else.

Same goes for life. For leadership. For love.

When you start with your own breath — your own nourishment, your own peace — you lead better. Love better. Live better.

Because from fullness, we give differently.

Fullness Isn't in the Volume — It's in the Depth

We've been conditioned to associate a full life with *big* energy. Packed calendars. Loud laughter. Busy rooms. Shiny wins. A sense of movement, noise, output — proof that something's *happening*.

But what if fullness isn't measured in volume... but in *depth*? In the way your breath softens when no one needs you. In the silence that feels safe, not awkward. In the moment you're fully immersed in something — not for the camera, not for a comment — but just for *you*.

There are entire lives happening quietly.

- Someone writing a story no one else will read
- Someone walking a trail without sharing a step of it
- Someone tending to a small, gentle joy — and never needing it to perform

This isn't shrinking.

This is sovereignty.

You don't need to be louder to be more alive. You don't need to be seen to be whole. Fullness is what happens when you let yourself *feel everything* —even in silence.

The Power of Quiet Confidence

There's a kind of confidence that doesn't announce itself. It doesn't need bold fonts or perfect reels. It doesn't need to take up space loudly. It just *exists* — in the way someone carries themselves when they're no longer trying to prove anything.

Quiet confidence isn't about shrinking. It's about not needing to *inflate*.

It's:

- The pause before you answer — because you're not rushing to impress
- The smile you don't need to post — because you know it was real
- The decision not to explain — because your "no" is enough

It's steady. It's self-sourced. It doesn't demand the spotlight — because it's already lit from within.

We've been sold the idea that confidence must be extroverted, assertive, loud. But confidence that's lived — not performed — radiates. You don't need to dial yourself up to be taken seriously. You don't need to perform energy to be worthy of the room.

Your groundedness *is* your presence.

The quieter you become…the more powerfully you're heard.

What It Means to Take Up Space Without Noise

You don't have to be loud to take up space. You don't have to dominate to be powerful. You don't have to perform to be real.

Taking up space isn't about volume — it's about *being*. Being grounded in a room without explaining yourself. Being visible without apologising. Being true — even when it's quiet, even when it's slow.

You can take up space by standing still. You can take up space with a pause, with a breath, with a boundary. You can lead with softness and still be felt.

We live in a culture that mistakes noise for leadership. But the most impactful people often say less — and live more. They don't need to fill the silence. They don't need to announce their worth. They just *are* — and that's enough.

This chapter isn't about disappearing. It's about no longer needing to decorate your presence with noise. You're allowed to be quiet.

And still take up all the space you need.

The Still Lake That Reflects Everything

A still lake doesn't rush. It doesn't crash against the shore or shout for attention. It simply holds. And in its stillness, it reflects the entire sky. Clouds pass. Light changes. Winds stir the surface — but the depth remains.

This is what a full life can look like.

Still. Present. Reflective. Whole.

You don't need to churn the water to prove you're alive. You don't need to be in motion to be meaningful. Like the lake, your calm can reveal what's real. Your depth can hold what words cannot. Your presence can invite others to soften, too.

We are drawn to the loud — until we've lived through enough

noise. Then we begin to crave what's *quiet*... and true. Let your life reflect what matters. Not with performance, but with peace. Stillness is not the absence of power.

It's the presence of *depth*.

Reflection — Where Have You Equated Noise with Worth?

Pause.
Breathe.
And ask yourself:

- When did visibility become the measure of value?
- When did volume start to equal power?
- When did you begin performing life, instead of living it?

This world rewards the loud. The fast. The seen. But that's not the only way to move through it. There is worth in stillness. There is strength in depth.

There is *you* — beneath the performance.

Journal Moment

- Where have you been measuring your life by visibility — likes, comments, applause — instead of meaning?
- What part of you is quietly craving depth, solitude, or sincerity — not attention?
- What would it feel like to live your day fully — even if no one saw it, liked it, or praised it?
- What do you long to experience — not post, not prove, but truly *feel*?

You don't have to be seen to be real. You don't have to be loud to be powerful. You don't have to perform to be alive. This is your permission to choose presence over performance. Truth over trend. Life over image.

Pause. Reflect. Realign.

Let the noise fall away. Your worth was never meant to be broadcast. It was meant to be lived.

And from here — you get to choose how.

Edge Move — Choose Depth Over Noise

This week, choose depth.

- Sit with one experience — fully.
- Resist the urge to share it. Just let it be *yours*.
- Say less in a conversation — and feel the power in your silence.
- Skip one performance. Do one thing with no proof, no post, no polish.
- Watch what softens in you when you stop trying to be *more*.

You don't have to chase attention. You don't have to narrate your life. You just have to *live it* — deeply, quietly, honestly.

And that is enough.

Chapter 5
Becoming the Mountain

"I realised that I don't have to be perfect. All I have to do is show up, and enjoy the messy, imperfect, and beautiful journey of my life."

— *Kerry Washington*

What It Means to Become the Mountain

For most of life, we're climbing. Striving for the next level. Reaching toward the next version of ourselves. Pushing, proving, performing.

There's nothing wrong with the climb. It teaches you grit. Grace. Perspective. But eventually, something shifts. You stop asking, *"What's the next peak?"* And start asking, *"What if I've already arrived?"*

That's when you become the mountain.

Still. Strong. Weathered.

No longer chasing approval — just rooted in your truth. You stop rushing toward meaning and start *holding it*. You stop performing power and start *being it*.

Becoming the mountain doesn't mean you have nothing left to learn. It means you know how to stand — with calm, with conviction, with no need to explain your elevation. This isn't the end of the journey. It's the moment you realise: you *are* the ground you stand on.

You're Not Rebuilding — You're Integrating

After a fall, a change, a diagnosis, a breakdown... the pressure is often to bounce back.

Rebuild. Reinvent. Rise.

But what if you don't need to *start again*? What if the power is in integrating — not replacing? You're not erasing the past. You're choosing what to carry forward. Not everything has to come with you. But not everything has to be thrown away, either.

You can:

- Keep the softness that survival taught you
- Hold the boundaries you learned the hard way
- Honour the ambition — but reshape the pace
- Take the lessons — without dragging the weight

You're not broken. You're not a blank slate. You're layered. Seasoned. Whole. The old story was striving. The new one is *sovereignty*. You're not becoming someone new.

You're finally becoming someone true.

You Don't Owe Anyone a Performance

You've spent years curating how you're seen. The calm professional. The strong one. The capable one. The one who keeps going. And maybe it served you — for a while.

But the mountain doesn't audition. It doesn't dress itself up to be believed. It doesn't explain its shape, its silence, or its stillness.

It simply *is*.

You are allowed to show up without packaging. Without small talk. Without spin. You are allowed to be a little quieter. A little slower. A little more you. You don't owe the world a version of yourself it finds easy to understand. You don't have to decorate your peace. You just have to live it.

And if people don't get it? That's okay. They'll adjust — or they won't.

But either way: *you're done performing.*

When You Know What's Yours, You Stop Grabbing at Everything

There was a time when we said yes because we didn't want to miss out. When we grabbed every opportunity — not because it lit us up, but because we didn't yet know what was *ours*. The climb teaches us ambition.

But the edge teaches us discernment.

And once we know what's truly ours — we stop chasing what isn't. You don't need to impress. You don't need to respond to every message. You don't need to outrun your own rhythm just to keep up with someone else's.

You start doing less — and owning it more.

Because **FOMO** (fear of missing out) only exists when you haven't fully claimed what you *already have*. The more grounded you become in your own life — your values, your pace, your version of success — the less you're pulled by the shimmer of other people's paths.

Choosing *not* to do something isn't weakness.

It's power.

It's presence.

It's the muscle of self-trust — saying, "This isn't for me. And I'm okay not being part of it."

When you become the mountain, you don't fear missing the view from someone else's summit.

You *are* the view.

When you stand like a mountain, your "no" is as rooted as your "yes." You trust your instincts. You don't rush to explain your energy. Because you know now - what's yours will meet you where you are —not just where you hustle.

You're Allowed to Take Up Space — Calmly, Fully, Quietly

There's a story many of us inherited: That to take up space, we must be loud. Commanding. Constantly proving.

But real presence doesn't demand attention. It simply holds its ground.

We are allowed to exist fully — without needing to justify the room we take. Without being the loudest. Without offering disclaimers. Without performing capability to be worthy of respect.

We're allowed to sit at the table in stillness. To show up without adjusting our edges. To be fully ourself — even if that self is quiet, soft, or evolving.

Mountains don't apologise for their outline. They don't shrink to fit the landscape. They don't need signage to announce their worth.

This isn't arrogance.

It's alignment.

You're not trying to take someone else's space.

You're finally owning your own.

The Tree Line Stops, But You Keep Going

Climbing a mountain, you eventually reach the tree line. It's the point where the trees stop growing — where the air thins, the path narrows, and everything gets quieter. There's less shade. Less noise. Less company. But also more sky.

The further you go, the fewer people come with you. And that can feel lonely — until you realise - you didn't come all this way to be surrounded.

You came to *see clearly*.

At the top, there's wind. Silence. Space. And a different kind of strength — not the kind that pushes through, but the kind that *knows when to stop and stand still*.

Before you become the mountain, you often summit a few. Not to prove something — but to gain perspective.

When I'm summiting a mountain, it's never comfortable. You're above the tree line. The shelter is gone. The wind hits harder up here — raw and unfiltered. It can be cold. Harsh. It's not a place you linger for long.

But what you *gain*?

Perspective.

You can see. Really see. All around you. A full 360 degrees. You don't have your usual comforts — but you do have clarity. Peace. Breath. And that moment — even if brief — reminds you what matters.

You climbed for a reason.

This is where you meet yourself — without noise, without mirrors, without performance. And you realise:

You don't need to climb anymore.

You are already where you were meant to be.

Not because it's perfect. There is no perfect. But because it's *you*.

Reflection — You've Become What You Were Seeking

Pause here. No striving. No fixing. Just truth.
You began this book looking for something —
Clarity.
Peace.
Strength.
Maybe just a quieter way of being in the world.
But somewhere along the way…you stopped searching outward. And started returning inward.

Journal Moment

- What do you need to let go of — fully, finally, for good?
- What has returned to you — stronger, clearer, or softer than before?
- Where in your life do you now feel most like yourself — unedited, grounded, whole?
- What parts of you no longer need to be explained, justified, or performed?

You're not who you were when you started this book. And you're not even trying to be. You've stopped climbing someone else's mountain. You've stopped chasing. You've stopped proving. And now — you've become the mountain.
Steady. Rooted. Unapologetically you.

Pause. Reflect. Realign.

This is the arrival. But it's also the beginning. You've become what you were seeking — not by adding more, but by returning to less. And now, you lead from within. From the edge.

From truth.

Edge Move — Stand Where You Are

This week, do nothing more than *stand*.

No pushing forward. No climbing to prove. No need to chase insight, approval, or momentum.

Just breathe. Be.

Stand in your presence.

Stand in your pace.

Stand in your clarity.

Stand in your softness.

Let the wind blow. Let others move past. Let the silence stay. You're not behind. You're not unfinished. You're not waiting to become.

You already are.

Part Two
Standing in the Space Between

Chapter 6
The Edge is Real

"You can be shattered, and then you can put yourself back together piece by piece. But what can happen over time is this: You wake up one day and realize that you have put yourself back together completely differently."

Glennon Doyle Melton

The Silent Shift

You don't always see it coming. There's no fanfare. No flashing sign. Sometimes, the moment your life begins to change sounds like a whisper. Or a sigh. Or a single thought you barely notice:

"This isn't it anymore."

The edge doesn't always arrive with drama. Sometimes, it looks like a perfectly normal Tuesday. You're making coffee. Scanning your inbox. Smiling on cue.

And yet — something's off. You feel strangely hollow in places that used to feel full. What once gave you energy now just... exists. And the mask you've been wearing? It's getting heavy.

This is the edge.

It's not a breakdown. It's not burnout. Not yet. It's the uncomfortable, undeniable knowing that something deep within you is shifting. And you can't ignore it forever. For a while, you might try. You'll talk yourself out of it. Say things like:

- *"I should be grateful."*
- *"It's just a busy time."*
- *"I'm probably just tired."*
- *"Everyone feels like this, right?"*
- *"It's the time of the month, yes?"*

But eventually, you realise the unease isn't going away. It's growing. Not to harm you — but to get your attention. Because you're standing at the edge of a life that doesn't quite fit anymore.

And the most courageous thing you can do... is stop pretending that it still does.

I remember standing at the kitchen counter, staring out the window. Nothing dramatic. Just a Wednesday, I think. Or maybe a Thursday. I honestly couldn't tell you. The moment wasn't significant enough to pin to a date.

But something didn't feel right.

Not wrong enough to call the doctor. Not sad enough to cry. Just... a shadow I couldn't name. Like a small cloud drifting across an otherwise clear sky — not enough to change the weather, but just enough to make me notice the shift in light.

I couldn't explain it. Couldn't put words to it. I just didn't feel quite right. Maybe I was hungry. I ate some toast and got on with my day.

But at the back of my mind, this disquiet stayed. Something in me whispered: *"Pay attention."* And two months later, I knew exactly why.

The Disguise of 'Fine'

We become experts at pretending. You learn to say *"I'm fine"* with a smile that doesn't quite reach your eyes. You fill your calendar so full that you can't hear your own thoughts. You show up, do the work, take care of others, hit the goals — and still wonder why you feel so far away from yourself.

Fine is a disguise. A socially acceptable smokescreen for "this isn't working anymore, but I don't know what to do about it." And the problem with *fine* is that it's hard to argue with. It doesn't throw red flags. It just quietly erodes you — one polite smile, one over-given yes, one ignored gut feeling at a time.

You might even be celebrated while you're fading. The awards keep coming. The clients keep clapping. The team keeps leaning on you. And inside, you're shrinking. Because we've been conditioned to equate performance with value.

If you're doing well, you *must* be well — right?

This Isn't It Anymore

There comes a moment — sometimes sudden, sometimes slow — when you stop negotiating with yourself. No more internal bartering:

"Just get through this week."
"Things will settle down next month."
"Maybe it's just my hormones."

At some point, you hit a truth so clear you can't reason your way around it anymore:

This isn't it.

It doesn't mean everything is wrong. That's what makes it confusing. On paper, things might even look great. You're doing what you always said you wanted. You've built something. You've achieved. You've arrived. But you don't feel *here*. You feel... gone. Or like you're only halfway inside your own life.

For me, that moment came with a to-do list.

I looked at the list of my most important jobs, and I thought - *really*? This is what I think matters today?" If I crumpled this paper up and just threw it away, would it matter? Would the world stop? Would my world stop? The answer was no. None of it really mattered.

It was a quiet but jarring moment of realisation: the things that used to define me no longer made sense. My list was full, but my life was hollow. And I couldn't unsee it. This wasn't a breakdown. It was a breakthrough in disguise. A moment of deep, inconvenient honesty — the kind that changes everything, if you let it.

Letting go didn't happen all at once. It never does. But from that moment on, I could feel the unravelling begin — not in a destructive way, but in a clarifying one. I wasn't falling apart. I was falling back to myself. You can be high-achieving and hollow. You can be functioning and floundering. You can be "fine" — and falling apart.

The edge often hides behind *fine*. But your body knows. Your joy knows. Your gut knows. And eventually, it starts to whisper louder.

Edges I've Witnessed

Once you've stood at your own edge, you start to see it everywhere. You recognise it in the pause before someone answers *"How are you?"* You hear it in the voice that's too bright, the laugh that comes too fast, the story that's too rehearsed.

And when you've been there — really been there — you know what it costs to hold it all together when something inside is quietly falling apart.

I've spoken with countless women and men who've stood at their edge. It rarely looks like chaos. It often looks… normal. Functional. Even successful.

The woman in the cereal aisle — overwhelmed by decision fatigue, walked out mid-shop.

The girl who got promoted, looked around her shiny new office, and realised she didn't recognise who she'd built this life for.

The one who received their divorce papers and felt only relief — realising they'd emotionally left that marriage long ago.

These weren't collapses. They were *clarities*. Edges disguised as everyday moments. That's the thing: the edge doesn't always arrive like a thunderclap. Sometimes, it shows up in a quiet conversation, a casual Sunday, or a single sentence you whisper in the dark:

"I don't want this anymore."

And when you finally let yourself hear it — really hear it — that's when the shift begins.

The Fear of Letting Go

We don't hold on because we love what is. We hold on because we're scared of what comes next. Letting go feels like freefall. It threatens everything we've built — or at least, everything we've *told ourselves* we've built.

We say things like:

- *"But I've invested so much time."*
- *"What if I regret it?"*

- *"Who am I if I'm not this?"*
- *"What will people think?"*

We tell ourselves that staying is safer — more responsible, more logical. But often, it's just more familiar. And the familiar — even when it's slowly draining us — can feel less terrifying than the unknown.

Letting go asks us to risk being misunderstood. To disappoint people we've spent years impressing. To change a story mid-sentence — without knowing how it ends. It's not just fear of failure. It's fear of unravelling. Fear of being seen without the roles, titles, or rhythms that once made us feel important or needed.

But here's what I've learned at the edge:
You can't evolve and cling at the same time.

There's no way to stretch into a new life while gripping the old one with white knuckles. Eventually, something has to loosen — and it's either your grip or your soul.

Why the Edge Isn't a Breakdown

We're so quick to label change as crisis. To assume that if something's cracking open, it must be falling apart. But what if you're not breaking down?

What if you're breaking *through*? What if this discomfort isn't dysfunction — it's direction? What if the ache isn't failure — it's friction between your truth and your current life?

The edge is not the end. It's a threshold. A hinge moment. A doorway disguised as doubt.

It often arrives after a long season of "coping."

You've adjusted. Endured. Managed. Minimized. But your soul knows the difference between surviving and actually living — and eventually, it speaks. Not in shouts. But in symptoms:

- Apathy where there used to be joy
- Rage that comes from nowhere
- A body that won't stop aching
- A gut feeling you can't ignore anymore

We've been taught to override those signs. To be strong. To push through. But real strength isn't pushing past your edge. It's *honouring* it.

Because the edge is where the performance stops.

It's where you stop striving to be impressive and start learning how to be honest. And from that honesty — your real leadership begins.

When You Stay Anyway

Sometimes, even after you know — you stay. You know this isn't it anymore. You've felt the tug, heard the whisper, seen the signs. But you keep showing up. Keep performing. Keep playing the part.

Why? Because staying is easier to explain than leaving. Because walking away from something good-but-wrong feels harder than surviving something awful. Because you've built a life that makes sense to everyone but you. And tearing that down — or even gently stepping back — feels like betrayal.

So you stay.

And you tell yourself:

- *"It's not that bad."*
- *"Other people have it worse."*
- *"I'll deal with it after this next project/term/year."*

You stay... until staying becomes its own kind of self-abandonment. The body will always tell the truth eventually.

Mine did. Loudly. And not in polite little hints — but in pain, fatigue, and a kind of numbness that no amount of yoga or coffee could fix.

When you stay past your truth, the cost compounds. Not because you're weak, but because your soul is smarter than your spreadsheet. You can't logic your way out of an edge. You have to feel your way through.

And sometimes, feeling it is what finally moves you.

The Turn Toward Truth

The moment you stop pretending is rarely loud. It's not a dramatic announcement or a grand reinvention. It's a breath. A pause. A quiet decision that sounds like:

"I'm not doing this to myself anymore."

Sometimes the first move isn't quitting the job or ending the relationship or changing your whole life. Sometimes, the first move is simply telling the truth — to yourself. You don't have to know what comes next. You don't have to have a five-year plan. You just have to stop gaslighting your own gut.

That's what the edge offers — a chance to meet yourself again — without the noise. Without the costume. Without the pressure to prove anything.

And in that moment, something beautiful begins.

Not a reinvention, exactly. More like a remembering. A remembering of who you were before the roles. Before the 'shoulds'. Before the performance.

The edge is where you drop the script. And begin writing something real.

"You can start over at any time. Every time you choose yourself, it's a new beginning."

— *Alexandra Elle*

Voice from the Edge

A friend told me about the moment she realised her soul had already made the decision — long before her mind caught up...

> *It was the automatic response I gave to someone's question that triggered 'my moment'. It held up a mirror to my very soul.*
>
> *"Are you going to apply?" They asked.*
>
> *"Absolutely not". I replied with such absolute certainty. The promotion was what I'd been working towards for years. Yet putting the shock of my automatic response aside, I knew with fierce certainty it was the right decision. However, it frightened me. When did I decide this wasn't my path? How long had I known? Why hadn't I realised before now?*
>
> *It was clear I was well down the road to burn out. Reflection helped me realise I was playing a key role in a circus and I needed to escape, quickly before it consumed me. But doing that would come at great cost.*
>
> *Accessing coaching helped me to untangle what was happening. Pausing and really listening to that internal quiet voice helped me see clearly. I found a way forward that, to some, looked brave, for others... foolish. Regardless I knew it was right.*
>
> *I went back to basics and re-established what mattered and who I was. What makes me tick, sparks joy and energy. For the first time in a long while I was able to articulate my core believes and values with clarity. It didn't matter what others thought... I knew without doubt that I had found my path.*
>
> *And with that, I found peace.*
>
> *— Sarah Gill*

The Cold Beach at Low Tide

The edge, to me, is like standing barefoot on a cold beach just as the tide recedes. At first, the water pulls away so gently you barely notice. But then the sea keeps going — pulling back, further than you expected. And suddenly, you're standing on wet sand that wasn't meant to be walked on.

It's uncomfortable. Exposed. The shells are sharp. The stones are slippery. You see things you didn't know were there — bits of memory, grief, restlessness, dreams you shelved ten years ago.

You're not drowning. But you're not on solid ground either. You're in-between. Between who you've been... and who you're becoming. You could turn back. Wrap yourself in the towel of your old life and pretend the tide never shifted.

Or you could stay. Barefoot. Bracing. Brave.

Because soon — not immediately, but eventually — the tide changes. And when it comes back in, it doesn't just pull away the old. It brings something new. The edge isn't a cliff.

It's a turning point.

Reflection: Where Are You Standing?

Take a breath. Be honest with yourself. This isn't about judgment. It's about truth — even if it's quiet. So much of life is shaped around appearances. We make things look fine. We keep the rhythm going. But underneath, something can feel off — and we keep going anyway.

This is your moment to pause. To look beneath the surface.

Not to fix. Just to notice.

Journal Moment

- Where in your life does everything *look* fine... but *feel* wrong?
- What truth have you been pushing down, explaining away, or scheduling over?
- Where are you performing strength... instead of honouring your edge?
- What would shift if you allowed honesty to lead, just a little more?

You don't have to rip it all up. You don't need to burn it all down. But you do need to stop pretending something works when it doesn't. Because even one moment of truth — one honest breath — can begin a whole new chapter.

Pause. Reflect. Realign.

Let's use this rhythm as a compass throughout the book.

Wherever you are on the path — you're allowed to stop and check if it still fits.

You don't need a crisis to realign. Just honesty.

Edge Move: Stop and Tell the Truth

This week, choose one area of your life where something isn't aligned — and name it. You don't need to fix it. You don't need to justify it. You just need to *say it*. To yourself, or to someone safe.

Try this sentence:

"I've been pretending this is fine, but it's not."

That's it. That's the move.

Andrea Ubhi

You don't need to leap — yet. But you've just stopped hiding. And that's where everything starts to shift.

Chapter 7
The Slow Burn

> "You can choose courage, or you can choose comfort, but you cannot choose both."
>
> *Brene Brown*

The Cost of Holding On

Letting go rarely begins with a dramatic moment. More often, it starts with a quiet sense of resistance. A small sigh, you don't explain. A reluctance to open your laptop. A thought like: *"I just need a bit more coffee. Then I'll feel normal."*

But normal doesn't come.

Instead, you get the slow burn. The low hum of fatigue. The edge of irritability. The calendar you designed... now feels like a trap. You're not unhappy. Not exactly. But something feels off — and has for a while.

You tell yourself it's a phase. A hormonal dip. The weather. You rationalise: *"I should be grateful. Look at everything I have."* And you are grateful.

But also? You're tired. Not sleepy. **Soul-tired.** This is the slow, creeping cost of holding on too long.

It doesn't shout. It just waits — quietly, patiently — for you to notice that you're operating on fumes.

You start avoiding small things. Then big ones. You fantasise about holidays, silence, and cancelling everything for a week. You long for space, but keep adding more.

* * *

I remember driving to work, turning off the car... and just sitting there. I didn't want to move. Nothing dramatic. No tears. Just a quiet, heavy pause.

Then I turned the car back on, drove around the block—as if that extra loop might change something—parked again, sighed, and got on with my day.

I told myself I just needed to wake up a bit more. Or that the weather was messing with me. And I did what most of us do. I brushed it off. Pushed through. Told myself I'd be fine.

* * *

We're told that life is hard. That we have to dig deep. That it's supposed to be difficult. Grin and bear it. Get on with it.

Everyone's tired. You're not special. So we carry on. Even when something doesn't feel right. Even when our bodies are trying to speak. Even when our minds are quietly fraying at the edges.

The cost of holding on is rarely loud.

But in hindsight? That moment was a sign. A subtle one. Easy to miss. But it was there. It's in the moments we ignore what we already know. This is how holding on looks in real life.

It's not always dramatic.

Sometimes, it just looks like scrolling on your phone in the bathroom, too depleted to rejoin your life. And yet, you keep going. Because that's what you do.

Until one day…the cost catches up.

What We're Really Holding

It's easy to look at your calendar and blame the exhaustion on logistics. Too many meetings. Too much admin. Too many hats, all balanced precariously on the same overstretched head.

But often, what's weighing us down isn't the *tasks*. It's what those tasks *represent*. We're not just holding diaries and deadlines.

We're holding:

- Identities we've outgrown
- Expectations we never consented to
- Roles we were praised for, so we kept them, long after they stopped fitting
- Other people's assumptions about what we're capable of, and whether we can "handle it all"

Sometimes we hold on because it's working… for everyone else. Because it's *convenient* for us to keep saying yes. Because we're the one who "just makes it happen." And it's become easier to keep performing than to pause and ask, *"Is this even what I want anymore?"*

Even the things we once *loved* can become heavy when they're piled too high, or when we're clinging out of habit rather than alignment.

And the tricky part? You can't put something down until you realise you're carrying it.

The Breaking Point

There was a time when I had three young children, two dental practices, a team of over forty, and was still working full clinical days. I was winning awards — Dentist of the Year, Cosmetic Pioneer of the Year. My diary was full. My reputation strong. My practice thriving.

On the surface, I was exactly where I'd aimed to be.

And I was in agony.

My back was screaming. I was exhausted all the time. Something was draining me — and in hindsight, it's obvious what it was: *everything*.

But I didn't have the time to unpack it. I couldn't afford to stop and analyse what was working and what wasn't — because that would just create *more* work.

So I did what most high-functioning humans do: I pushed through. But here's the thing about tunnels. Eventually, you have to get out. And that means being brave enough to stop and ask: *What's actually going on here?*

Planning your way out takes more energy in the short term. But it saves your soul in the long run. So, I started thinning my life down. I sold one of my practices — a process that took over a year.

And then I asked myself a question I'd never dared to ask before:

What if my body is trying to save me? Because by then, the back pain was constant. I laughed, genuinely, as I realised — *how much louder could my body scream?*

So I listened.

And I stopped doing clinical dentistry. It was one of the most pivotal decisions of my life. The title I'd carried for 25 years — gone. The label, the rhythm, the identity — all released.

And what followed was... space. And the question:

If I'm not "Andrea the dentist," who am I now?

Not everyone understood. Questions were asked. But here's what I know: This is my life.

And I don't need anyone's permission to live it differently.

What Holding On Too Long Looks Like

Not all burnout looks like lying on the floor in dramatic fashion.

Sometimes, it's sneakier.

Holding on too long doesn't always feel like a breakdown. Sometimes, it just looks like… your normal life, but slightly more unbearable than it used to be.

Here are a few signs you might be holding on past your edge:

- You feel slightly resentful of everyone who expects something from you… which is, unfortunately, everyone.
- You fantasise about cancelling everything and running off to a beach shack with no WiFi.
- You scroll Pinterest looking at yurts.
- You keep saying, *"Next month things will calm down,"* and you've been saying that for 5 years.
- You feel weirdly jealous of people who've quit their careers to become potters, yoga teachers, or goat farmers.
- You do absolutely everything — and still feel like you've done nothing.
- You've booked things into your diary and secretly hope they get cancelled.
- You wake up tired, go to bed wired, and call caffeine self-care.

And yet… you keep going. Because people rely on you.

Because you're "good at it." Because it's easier than explaining why you need to stop.

This isn't about failure. This is about honesty. Sometimes, the most loving thing you can do for your work, your people, and yourself is to say:

This isn't working anymore. And that matters.

Why We Stay

We stay because it used to work. Because once, this role, this rhythm, this life lit us up — and it's hard to let go of something that was once right, even if it no longer is.

We stay because people count on us. Because we've built things — businesses, careers, families — and there's pride in what we've created. Because walking away from something that looks successful on the outside can feel like failure… even when it's freedom.

We stay because we don't want to disappoint anyone. Because we fear being labelled ungrateful, dramatic, unreliable, selfish.

We stay because we've invested so much — and surely, we should see it through. And then there's the trickiest one:

We stay because we're good at it. When you're good at something, the world gives you very little incentive to stop doing it. But "good at it" isn't the same as aligned. Or energised. Or well.

There's a strange internal guilt that comes from even *considering* letting go of something that's still technically working. Especially if others would be thrilled to be in your shoes.

"Who do you think you are to step back from this?"
"Some people would kill for your life."
"You should be grateful."

You can be grateful — and done. You can love what you've built — and still feel called to shift. Staying isn't always wrong. But staying out of fear, guilt, or autopilot can slowly chip away at your joy.

Sometimes the braver thing isn't to keep holding on. It's to recognise the moment you're ready to set something down.

Identity Unravelling

Letting go of a role isn't just a career decision. It's an identity shift.

When I stepped back from clinical dentistry, I didn't just stop doing smile makeovers and dental veneer cases. I let go of the title I'd carried for decades — the label people introduced me with, the foundation of my confidence, the thing I knew I was good at.

It wasn't a clean break. It was disorienting. At first, I felt like I'd lost something solid. Like I was unmoored. When someone asked what I did, I stumbled. Was I still a dentist if I wasn't doing dentistry?

This is the part most people don't talk about:

The strange grief that can come with stepping out of a role — even one that was slowly draining you.

Because when we let go of the label, we also let go of:

- The predictable rhythm
- The automatic credibility
- The familiar story we tell ourselves about who we are

And without that, there's a space. An awkward, wobbly space where something new might grow — but for a while, it's just empty.

You might question everything. Am I still ambitious? Am I wasting my potential? Who am I if I'm not *that* anymore? But here's what I've learned:

That space isn't emptiness. It's possibility. It's where your next chapter begins — the one that's not written in reaction to others' expectations.

It's where you meet yourself again — not as a title, but as a whole human.

Letting Go as a Brave Act

Let's be clear: letting go is not giving up. It's choosing truth over performance. Alignment over applause. Courage over comfort.

Walking away from something that's *almost* right — but not quite — is far braver than sticking it out because it's what's expected.

Real bravery often doesn't look heroic. It looks like an email drafted but not sent. A conversation you finally start. A diary block that says *nothing at all* — and stays that way.

I've seen it over and over again in those I work with:

- A practice principal who sold her practice to get her soul back
- A dentist who dropped her five-day week to start writing again
- A mum who stopped volunteering for everything and finally slept
- A woman who walked away from a toxic friendship and said, "That counts too."

Letting go doesn't always mean leaving the job or moving house or selling everything you own. Sometimes, it starts with just saying: *"This isn't serving me anymore."*

That moment — that decision — is a hinge. It's the moment you stop asking, *"How do I keep up?"* And start asking, *"What would feel honest now?"* And that question?

It's the one that leads you home.

The Shift That Follows

When you finally let go of what no longer fits — there's usually a pause. Not a fanfare. Not instant clarity. Just… space. Sometimes uncomfortable, often quiet, and surprisingly peaceful. You might not feel triumphant at first. You might feel unsure. There may even be guilt:

Shouldn't I be doing more? Shouldn't I feel more productive?

You've been so used to chasing, managing, holding, proving — that the absence of all that can feel like laziness. But it's not.

It's healing.

That space you've created? That's where clarity has a chance to speak. You start noticing things again. The way your body feels when it's not bracing. The creativity that returns when you're not buried. The flickers of joy, curiosity, and energy that feel almost… unfamiliar.

For me, the shift didn't arrive all at once. But gradually, I noticed I could breathe deeper.

I enjoyed my work again. I felt more present with my family. I started spending more time outdoors — not as an escape, but as an expression of freedom.

And perhaps most importantly: I began to enjoy who I was becoming. Not because I was doing more. But because I was finally doing *me*.

Letting go created space. And in that space, I didn't disappear — I returned. Not to the woman I used to be…

But to the one I'd been growing into all along.

> **"She remembered who she was, and the game changed."**
> — Lalah Delia

Letting Go

Holding on too long is like gripping the side of a sinking raft. Your arms ache. Your shoulders burn. You're soaked, exhausted, tense. You think your grip is what's keeping you safe. But really, it's what's making you suffer.

It's not the river that's exhausting you —it's how tightly you're clinging.

You can't see where the current is going, so you grip harder. You whisper, *"Just a bit longer..."* But the longer you cling, the more you forget: you were built to float.

Letting go doesn't mean abandoning hope. It means loosening your grip. Trusting that your life can hold you. That your instincts are stronger than your fear.

That maybe — just maybe — it's safe to let the river carry you somewhere new.

Letting go feels risky.

But clinging to a sinking raft? That's a guaranteed way to drown.

Reflection: What Are You Still Carrying?

There are things we carry long after they've stopped serving us. Roles that once made sense. Routines that once felt good. Expectations we never agreed to, but perform anyway.

We carry them because they've become part of our identity. Or because we're afraid of what might happen if we put them down. But here's the truth: you're allowed to release what's become too heavy.

Even just for a moment.

Even just to see how it feels.

Journal Moment

- What are you still holding that no longer serves you — a role, a responsibility, a rhythm?
- What would it feel like to set it down, even temporarily?
- Where are you going through the motions in something you no longer believe in?
- If no one were watching — no judgment, no consequences — what would you let go of today?

You don't have to figure it all out. You don't have to fix it overnight. But naming it? That's where the release begins.

Pause. Reflect. Realign.

Let this be your cue to lighten the load — not by force, but by truth. The edge doesn't demand reinvention. It just asks you to stop pretending it's not time for change.

Edge Move: The Gentle Release

Choose one thing this week to *not hold*. It could be a task you've outgrown. A meeting you no longer need to attend. An identity you're ready to loosen your grip on.

Say no. Delegate. Cancel. Delay. Or simply tell someone close to you: *"I'm not going to keep carrying this."*

You don't need to justify it. You don't need to over-explain. You just need to begin.

Small releases make space for big returns.

Chapter 8

The Illusion of Control

> "One of the most calming and powerful actions you can do to intervene in a stormy world is to stand up and show your soul. Struggling souls catch light from other souls who are fully lit up and willing to show it."
>
> — Clarissa Pinkola Estés

Control Looks Like Safety (But it Isn't)

There's something delicious about a colour-coded calendar. Or a packing list made three weeks in advance. Or a meal plan that fits perfectly into a spreadsheet.

Control feels safe. Predictable. Efficient. It gives us the illusion that if we can *just get everything lined up*, nothing bad will happen.

If we prepare well enough, work hard enough, care deeply enough — surely we can avoid disappointment.

We don't call it fear. We call it being *organised, high-achieving, on top of things*. We even get praised for it. But underneath it?

Control is often just our brain's attempt to feel safe in a world that isn't.

It starts with the small things:

- Double-checking the email
- Booking the backup just in case
- Rewriting the to-do list because the font didn't feel right.

And before you know it, you're trying to manage everything — the plans, the people, the outcomes, the weather.

That's the crack in the armour: when something tiny goes wrong and you feel like the whole day is falling apart. That's not just frustration. That's your nervous system revealing how hard it's been working to hold everything together.

Control works... until it doesn't. Until the spreadsheet breaks. Until the body breaks. Until life — being life — doesn't go to plan.

And that's when we're invited to shift from managing everything... to trusting ourselves in anything.

What Control Is Really About

Control is rarely about the thing we say it's about. It's not really about the calendar, or the plan, or the fact that someone didn't reply to your email within 45 minutes.

Control is often fear in disguise. Fear of uncertainty. Fear of things going wrong. Fear of looking unprepared. Fear of being caught off guard. Fear of being disappointed — again.

It makes sense, really. Control gives us something to *do* when life feels unpredictable. It makes us feel useful. Competent. Strong. And in a world that can be chaotic, grief-filled, overwhelming... control is something we can cling to when we don't know what else to hold.

But here's the thing:
Control doesn't stop bad things from happening.
It just makes us think we're responsible when they do. It convinces us that if we'd just tried harder, planned better, worked later — we could have prevented the disappointment. It keeps us in hypervigilance. Busy. Tense. Braced. Constantly scanning for what might go wrong — and believing that if it does, it's our fault.

Control promises safety.

But often, it just gives us pressure. And the more we grip, the more we disconnect — from our bodies, our instincts, our peace.

True power isn't controlling everything.

It's learning to trust yourself, even when you can't.

The Myth of "If I Work Hard Enough…"

We're raised on a powerful idea — if you work hard enough, plan well enough, care deeply enough — things will go your way.

Effort = results.
Discipline = safety.
Hard work = control.

It's comforting, in theory. But in real life? You can do everything "right" — and things still fall apart. You can care deeply — and still get hurt. You can plan meticulously — and still have it unravel.

Hard work is valuable. Of course it is. But it isn't a guarantee. It doesn't protect you from grief, loss, rejection, or the human messiness of other people's choices. And yet, when things go wrong, what do we do? We double down.

- Rewrite the process.
- Add more systems.
- Blame ourselves for not anticipating the unexpected.

It's exhausting — and it never ends.

This myth — that if you just try hard enough, you can outrun discomfort — is a setup. It keeps us performing strength instead of practicing trust. It keeps us busy... but brittle. And it teaches us that rest is weakness, rather than wisdom.

True power isn't found in perfect preparation.

It's found in your ability to adapt, to stay open, to respond with clarity even when the outcome is uncertain. That's leadership. That's maturity. That's freedom.

When Control Becomes the Cage

Control feels empowering — until it starts controlling *you*. What begins as a clever way to manage life soon becomes the very thing that traps you.

- You micromanage your diary, then feel strangled by it.
- You optimise every process, then resent how rigid your systems have become.
- You make every decision, then wonder why you feel so alone.
- You carry everything — then collapse under the weight.

The problem with control is that it keeps *expanding*. Once you start trying to manage everything, there's no end to what you could be tweaking, perfecting, or anticipating. And here's the catch: the more tightly you hold the reins, the less space there is for other people to step in — or step up.

The very thing meant to keep you safe... begins to limit you. Your world gets smaller. Tighter. More brittle. And one day you realise — you're not in control. You're in a cage you built with good intentions. A beautiful, high-functioning, gold-plated cage — but a cage all the same.

Letting go doesn't mean losing power.

It means reclaiming it from the things that no longer deserve to hold it.

What It Costs Us

We don't always realise what control is costing us — until we stop. Because while it might look like things are "working," control often comes at the expense of things we value even more:

- **Trust.** When you grip too tightly, it sends a message — to your team, your family, even yourself — that no one else can be trusted to handle it.
- **Presence.** You're so busy managing the next ten steps, you miss the moment you're in.
- **Creativity.** When everything's pre-planned, there's no room for spontaneous brilliance.
- **Ease.** Even simple days feel tight and effortful.
- **Rest.** Control doesn't switch off. And neither do you.

And then there's **joy** — possibly the quietest casualty.

Control flattens joy. It makes fun feel inefficient. It makes relaxation feel irresponsible. It squeezes life into a box that's safe but sterile.

"I never feel more anxious than when I'm trying to get everything right."

— Probably Every Woman I've Coached, Ever.

You might look calm on the outside — but on the inside? You're spinning plates. Juggling flaming torches. Bracing for impact. And the truth is — you weren't built to live like that. You weren't meant to manage your way through life. You were meant to experience it. To shape it. To respond to it with wisdom, not white-knuckle control.

There's a cost to gripping everything.

And eventually, the invoice comes due — in your health, your spirit, or your spark.

The Shift to Trust

Letting go of control doesn't mean giving up. It means *trading force for flow*. It means shifting from the question: *"How do I manage everything?"*

To: *"What can I trust right now?"*

Trust doesn't mean everything will go to plan. It means *you'll be OK even if it doesn't*. This is where true leadership begins — not in hyper-efficiency, but in *calm responsiveness*.

It's not passive. It's powerful.

Because when you begin to trust:

- Yourself
- Your process
- Your team
- Your timing
- Even the hard days

...You create more space. And in that space, you lead better, love better, and live lighter.

I didn't stop being responsible when I let go of control. I became more discerning. I stopped trying to micromanage every outcome and started listening more closely to my instincts. I delegated — not just tasks, but trust.

And the world didn't collapse. In fact, it rose to meet me.

Letting go allowed others to step in. It gave my team room to grow. It gave my nervous system a rest. And it gave me back a deeper kind of confidence — one that didn't need everything to go perfectly to feel steady.

That's the kind of leadership I believe in. The kind that holds space, not tension.

What Opens Up When We Let Go

The surprising thing about letting go of control is not what you lose — but what you finally make space to *gain*. Because control fills every corner of your day with doing, checking, anticipating. When you release even a little of it… air rushes in.

Suddenly, you notice:

- You breathe deeper
- You interrupt less
- You sleep better
- You trust your team more
- You laugh — properly, not performatively
- You give things room to unfold, and realise most of them still work just fine without your constant interference.

When I let go of micro-managing my business, my team stepped into more ownership. When I stopped trying to pre-plan every outcome, creative solutions surfaced that I *never* would've scripted. When I stopped running my life like a military operation, I rediscovered joy. And time. And myself.

Letting go didn't make me weaker.

It made me lighter. And in that lightness, I became more present — which made me a stronger leader, partner, and human.

Letting go doesn't mean chaos.

It means clarity — the kind that arrives when you stop doing *everything* and start doing *what matters*.

From Control to Confidence

Control says: *"I must prevent everything from going wrong."*
  Confidence says: *"I trust myself to respond if it does."*
  This is the shift.
  Control is based on fear — the fear that something will fall apart if you're not gripping every detail.
  Confidence is based on self-trust — the belief that you're resourceful enough to handle what comes. Confidence doesn't need everything to go to plan. It doesn't panic at the unknown. It doesn't need to be the smartest or the most prepared in the room. It simply *knows who it is* — and responds from there.
  Here's what I've noticed in women who let go of control and start trusting themselves more:

- They interrupt less — because they're not trying to prove their value
- They delegate more — because they know their worth isn't in how much they do
- They lead calmly — because they're not operating from panic
- They get more done — because they're not busy second-guessing everything.

And here's the real magic:
Confidence spreads.
  When you lead from a place of inner steadiness, people feel it. They rise to meet it. They relax around it. They trust you — not because you control them, but because you don't need to.
  Confidence isn't – I wonder if they will like me. Confidence is –I like me, and that's enough.
  Letting go of control isn't passive. It's powerful.

It says — *I am not defined by what I manage. I am defined by how I show up.*

And when you show up calm, clear, and centred — everything changes.

The Tightly Held Rope

Imagine you're in a tug of war with life. You're gripping the rope with both hands, digging in your heels, pulling with everything you've got. You're tired. Blistered. Bracing for the next jolt.

But you keep holding on — because that's what strong people do, right? You're convinced that if you just pull harder, you'll win. The tension will ease.

But it doesn't. It tightens.

And the longer you hold, the more your hands burn. The more your shoulders ache. The more you resent the rope itself — even though it was *you* who picked it up. Then something strange happens.

You let go. Just a little. Maybe you loosen your grip. Maybe you take one hand off. Maybe, finally, you drop the rope completely.

And you don't fall. You don't lose. You stand. Lighter. Clearer. Unburned. Because the truth is — the rope wasn't keeping you upright and steady.

You were.

And you still are.

Voice from the Edge

One friend shared this story with me, and I think many of us will recognise ourselves in her words — that moment where stuckness feels safer than risk, and the first brave choice is simply movement.

"I remember feeling anxious, unsettled — like I'd lost all sense of focus and self-belief. Every decision felt like a question I couldn't answer. My thoughts were tangled, like spaghetti strands pulled in every direction, knotted and knotted again.

I stayed still. Stuck. Not because I wanted to — but because doing nothing felt safer than risking rejection. I told myself: at least here, I can't fail. But the truth? I was miserable.

It felt like I was stuck in a washing machine cycle — spinning, churning, and going nowhere. Was it hormonal? Physical? Maybe. But I knew the bigger issue was this 'fake safe zone' I'd built around myself.

And one day, I'd had enough.

Change is possible — but only when it's self-driven. I had to challenge the patterns that were keeping me stuck. Say: No more. I started small. Made a list. Created a little structure. Set one or two goals — not big ones. Just manageable things that gave me a sense of movement.

And slowly, that movement became momentum. I started to believe in myself again. Not all at once. But enough. Enough to keep going. Enough to feel proud of every small step. Enough to say — I'm changing this.

One choice at a time."

A friend, from the edge of her own change

Reflection: What Are You Still Gripping?

Take a breath. And be honest. Sometimes we hold on tightly — not because it's working, but because we're afraid of what might happen if we let go.

We grip timelines, expectations, outcomes, identities. We grip because it feels safer than trusting. We grip because we've been told that to be strong is to be in control.

But real strength doesn't live in tension.

It lives in trust.

Journal Moment

- Where in your life are you holding on too tightly — to people, roles, outcomes, timelines?
- What are you trying to control that can't actually be controlled?
- What's it costing you — energy, ease, trust, sleep, joy?
- What would it feel like to loosen your grip… just a little?

This isn't about letting everything go. It's not about becoming passive or careless. It's about releasing the illusion that control equals safety — and remembering that sometimes, the stronger move is to soften.

Pause. Reflect. Realign.

Let your grip soften. Let trust return in small, quiet ways. And notice what else becomes possible when your hands — and your heart — aren't so tightly clenched.

Edge Move: The Rope Drop

This week, choose one thing to let go of — not entirely, but lightly.

- A conversation you've been rehearsing
- A result you've been obsessing over
- A task you've been hovering around.

Step back. Loosen your grip. Watch what happens. Say to yourself:

"I don't need to manage this to be safe. I trust myself to respond, whatever comes."

That's leadership. That's power. That's how you stop performing control — and start living in calm confidence.

Chapter 9
The Quiet Voice Within

That Feeling You Keep Brushing Off

Y ou know the feeling. It's not dramatic. It doesn't shout. It arrives quietly — like a flicker. A breath. A small pause in your chest that whispers:
Something's not quite right.

You can't explain it. There's no data. No logic. Just a sense. So, naturally... you ignore it. You brush it off. Blame it on hormones, or tiredness, or being "too sensitive." You carry on. You say yes. You talk yourself out of it — because nothing's *actually wrong*, right?

But that's the thing about the quiet voice: it often speaks before anything looks off. It lives in the gap between your calendar and your gut. Between "this makes sense" and "this feels wrong."

I remember once hiring someone whose CV was excellent. The interview went well. The team all gave the thumbs up. On paper, the candidate was perfect. But something in me wasn't convinced. I couldn't explain it. It wasn't loud. Just… off.

I ignored the feeling.

We hired them. And it turned out to be a bad hire. Not because they weren't capable — but because they didn't share our core values. The signs were there. I just didn't listen.

Not a disaster — just one of those situations where, in hindsight, I knew. I didn't listen to my gut. And that quiet knowing? It had been there all along.

* * *

That feeling? It's the edge of your inner knowing. Not loud. Not obvious. But present. And when we override it too often, something strange happens: It stops speaking as clearly. Or worse — we stop believing it when it does.

But here's the truth — your inner voice isn't broken. It's just been buried under years of "shoulds" and "musts" and "you're being irrational." This chapter is about unearthing it — gently. So you can start hearing what you already know.

Why We Stop Listening

We're born knowing how to listen to ourselves. Hungry? We cry. Tired? We lie down wherever we are. Overstimulated? We walk away or shout about it. But over time, we learn to override those instincts.

We're praised for being agreeable, polite, easy to work with. We're told to sit still, be nice, follow instructions. We're taught that *thinking things through* is better than *feeling things through.*

By the time we're adults, we're fluent in strategy and second-guessing — but we've forgotten how to trust our own internal signals. Especially if we've been praised for being high-achieving, competent, calm under pressure — we get even better at ignoring ourselves. Because being intuitive starts to feel... inconvenient.

We outsource decisions to spreadsheets, checklists, coaches, mentors. We Google everything. We crowdsource answers we already have inside us — just to feel safer.

The world rewards logic.

But your inner knowing doesn't speak in logic. It speaks in sensation. In stillness. In that strange moment where something feels off, even though everything looks fine.

And if you've spent years overriding it, that's not a personal flaw. It's a survival strategy. You learned to tune out your inner voice because the world taught you to value certainty, productivity, and approval more than quiet wisdom.

But the voice is still there.

And it will speak again — especially if you slow down long enough to hear it.

The Signs Are Subtle — But They're There

Your inner knowing doesn't arrive like a marching band. It rarely demands attention. More often, it makes quiet suggestions — the kind that are easy to miss when you're moving fast.

The signs are subtle:

- A slight tightness in your chest before you say "yes"
- A weird resistance to opening a certain email
- A task you keep putting off, even though it's "important"
- That strange joy when someone cancels plans and you feel... relief
- A flicker of dread when you see a name on your phone

These are not problems to solve. They're signals to notice.

They whisper things like:

- *"You're pushing too hard."*
- *"You're pretending to be fine."*
- *"This isn't aligned anymore."*
- *"You don't need to go."*
- *"You're allowed to change your mind."*

And if we're honest, we *do* hear them — just briefly. But then we override them with logic, responsibility, or people-pleasing reflexes.

The body knows.

Before the mind rationalises. Before the spreadsheet says yes. Before the world claps and says, *"Well done."* That quiet voice inside doesn't need to explain itself. Its job isn't to justify — it's to *guide*. And when you stop brushing off the small signs?

You start making decisions that feel right *without needing a reason*.

I used to think I should squash the feelings that came with PMT — that they weren't real. That I should push them down and carry on. But then I grew up. I realised those feelings were often *exaggerated versions of the truth*. Things I'd been tolerating suddenly felt intolerable — and that wasn't irrational. That was insight.

So I stopped suppressing and started harnessing.

I began using that time of the month as fuel. I'd walk into the practice, stand at reception with my team and say, *"I've got PMT — so today, we're going to make some changes."*

And we would.

Policies would get reviewed. Systems would get overhauled.

Conversations that needed to happen — did. I stopped apologising for the edge in me.

I started trusting it instead.

Inner Knowing vs Fear, Ego, and Habit

One of the most common questions I hear is:

"But how do I know if it's my intuition… or just fear?"

It's a good question. Because not every inner voice is wisdom. Some are just… noise. Here's how they differ:

Fear is loud. Urgent. Panicked. It tells you to act fast. Or hide. Or fix something *right now*. It doesn't like risk, change, or unknowns.

Fear says:

"Don't do it, you'll fail."

"Stay small, stay safe."

"You're not ready."

Ego is defensive. Status-obsessed. It wants to be right, admired, needed. It hates being wrong, embarrassed, or overlooked.

Ego says:

"They'll think you're better than them."

"You can't quit now — what will people say?"

"You need to prove yourself."

Habit is automatic. Convenient. It keeps you on autopilot, doing things the way you always have — not because they feel right, but because they're *familiar*.

Habit says:

"This is just how I am."

"I've already invested too much."
"It's fine. It's always been fine."

Inner Knowing is different. It's calm. It doesn't rush. It doesn't shout. It doesn't bargain or perform.

Inner knowing says:
"This isn't right."
"You don't need a reason."
"It's time."
"You already know."

The voice of fear comes from the mind. The voice of wisdom comes from the body. If you're unsure which voice you're hearing — pause. Breathe.

Ask:
"Is this voice rooted in love or fear?"
"Is this familiar discomfort or genuine misalignment?"
"If I slowed down, what would I hear underneath the noise?"

With practice, you'll learn to tell the difference. And once you start honouring the quiet voice — the *real* one — it gets louder.

What My Gut Told Me (and I Ignored)

I've ignored my gut more times than I can count. Sometimes it was small — like saying yes to a dinner when my whole body said no. Sometimes it was bigger — like agreeing to a project that looked great on paper, but felt heavy before it even began. It looked great on paper. But I had that *feeling*.

You know the one.

Nothing's *wrong*, but you feel yourself tense. You rationalise, of course. Tell yourself not to be negative. And then later — sometimes weeks, sometimes months — you find yourself thinking — *"I knew it."*

And here's what I've realised:

Every time I override my inner knowing to be "sensible" or "nice" or "professional" — I pay for it twice. First, when I ignore it. And again, when it proves itself right.

The cost isn't just in outcomes. It's in the erosion of self-trust. Each time we betray our knowing, it gets harder to recognise it next time. And each time we honour it — even in tiny ways — we rebuild our relationship with it.

The gut doesn't need to be dramatic.

It just needs to be heard.

Learning to Listen Again

If you've spent years ignoring your intuition — you're not broken. You're human. And you can learn to listen again.

For me, it started in small ways. Saying no to something minor — just because it didn't feel right. Taking an extra day to make a decision — even when people wanted an answer *now*. Pausing before replying. Noticing when I tensed up… and asking why.

Intuition doesn't scream. It whispers. And the more noise in your life — the harder it is to hear it. So I created a bit more space. Less back-to-back meetings. Fewer outside opinions. More walks. More quiet.

And in that quiet, I noticed things:

- A contraction in my body before agreeing to something
- A strange energy drop in certain conversations
- That slight inner glow when something *was* aligned

It wasn't always comfortable. Sometimes, my inner voice said things I didn't want to hear.

Like:

"This relationship is draining you."
"You're doing this for approval, not joy."
"That title no longer fits."

But it also said:

"You're allowed to rest."
"That was brave."
"You already know the answer."

Learning to listen again wasn't a grand epiphany. It was dozens of small, quiet choices. Until one day, that quiet voice felt less like a stranger — and more like home.

What Happens When You Trust It

Trusting your intuition doesn't always feel good in the moment. It can feel disruptive. Unpopular. Like stepping off the well-lit path and walking into fog with only your instincts to guide you.

But here's what I've learned — that quiet voice? It rarely leads you somewhere *comfortable* — but it *always* leads you somewhere true.

There have been decisions I couldn't explain at the time — only that they felt right. And looking back, they changed everything.

- Saying no to a "dream" opportunity because it didn't feel aligned
- Leaving a role that looked perfect on paper
- Ending a friendship that had quietly expired
- Taking a creative risk that led to something unexpected — and good

Was it tidy? No. Did it make sense to everyone else? Definitely not. Did it feel true? Absolutely.

And that feeling — of doing the right thing for *you*, not for optics or logic or applause — is one of the deepest forms of calm I've ever known. Not instant relief. But a quiet certainty. A knowing that you're exactly where you're supposed to be — even if the map isn't clear yet. That's the thing about trusting your intuition — it doesn't always lead to easy.

But it always leads to real.

Turning Down the Noise

Your inner knowing isn't gone. It's just crowded out by noise. Noise from the outside — the opinions, advice, scrollable lives. And noise from the inside — the overthinking, the pressure, the perfectionism. To hear your intuition again, you don't need to try harder. You need to turn the volume down.

Here's what helps:

1. White Space

- Don't book every hour.
- Leave breathing room between tasks, meetings, days.
- Your insight often arrives *after* the doing stops.

2. Less Input

- Limit screens, podcasts, opinions.
- It's hard to hear yourself when everyone else is shouting.

3. Body First

- If your body contracts — pause.
- If it opens — listen.
- Notice your breath. Shoulders. Jaw.
- Your body tells the truth before your brain catches up.

4. Journal Without a Plan

- No prompt. No filter.
- Just pen on paper.
- Let your thoughts wander until something feels true.

5. Give It 24 Hours

- If you feel pressured to say yes — wait.
- If it's right today, it'll still be right tomorrow.

You don't need to do all of these. Try one. See what shifts. You might be surprised how quickly that quiet voice returns — not because you chased it... but because you *made space* for it.

Stillness is where we meet ourselves again.

Fog Clearing Just Enough to See One Step

Your inner knowing isn't a searchlight. It doesn't illuminate the whole path. It doesn't come with a map, a 10-year plan, or a guaranteed outcome. It's more like mist lifting just enough to see *one next step*.

That's it. You take that step — and the fog lifts a little more. Then a little more. And soon, you realise: the path was never fully clear. But it was always walkable.

That's how intuition works.

It rarely tells you everything. It just tells you enough. Enough to move. Enough to shift. Enough to trust the nudge without needing the narrative. You might want certainty. But what you *need* is direction.

And that's exactly what the quiet voice offers — one step at a time. No drama. No fireworks.

Just presence. Just guidance. Just next.

Reflection: What's Your Inner Voice Saying?

Take a moment. No pressure. No performance. Just presence. There's a voice inside you that knows. Not the noisy one shaped by other people's expectations. Not the fear voice or the productivity voice. The knowing one. The quiet one. The one that doesn't need to shout to be true.

You've heard it before — in the pit of your stomach, the tightness in your chest, the sudden resistance to something that "should" feel fine. But life gets loud. And often, we override that knowing to stay liked, approved, or on track.

Journal Moment

- When was the last time you knew, deep down… but ignored it?
- What did your body try to tell you — with tightness, tiredness, or resistance?
- Where are you crowding out your own voice with noise, advice, or obligation?
- If everything else went quiet, what would your knowing say right now?

You don't have to act on it yet. You don't have to make a grand change. You just have to notice — and honour that something in you still knows.

Pause. Reflect. Realign.

The most powerful decisions don't always begin in the mind. Sometimes they begin in a whisper. Your job isn't to force clarity. It's to make space for it.

Edge Move: Follow the Whisper

This week, choose one decision — big or small — and don't overthink it. Don't outsource it. Don't explain it. Just feel it.

Notice your body. Your breath. Your resistance. Your ease. And when you hear the whisper — follow it. Say to yourself: *"I already know."*

Because you do.

You always have.

Chapter 10
Letting the Old Burn

When You Know It's Time

There comes a moment when you just can't do it anymore. Not because you're failing. Not because you're weak. But because something in you has shifted — and the life you've built no longer fits the shape of who you are.

It might not be a dramatic collapse. It might just be a quiet ache. A sigh before opening your laptop. A strange feeling of detachment in a room where you used to feel energised. A thought that sneaks in when you're driving: *"This isn't it anymore."*

That thought?

That's the spark. Sometimes you ignore it. You tell yourself: *"It's just a phase."* You double down. Work harder. Push through. But the knowing doesn't leave. It lingers. It waits. And then one day — it speaks louder: *"You've outgrown this."*

This isn't about being ungrateful. It's about being honest. You're not walking away from your life. You're walking back to yourself.

And that begins not with adding something new — but with letting the old burn.

The Fire as Clarifier

Burning something down sounds dramatic. But sometimes, it's the only way to see what really matters. Fire strips away the excess. It doesn't ask for permission. It doesn't apologise.

It clears. It reveals.

And when you're willing to let something burn — an old role, a title, a way of living that no longer fits — you stop rearranging the clutter and start *clearing the path*.

This isn't chaos. It's clarity.

Because when the noise, the obligations, the expectations, and the people-pleasing are gone — what's left? What's true. What's solid. What was always yours.

The fire doesn't destroy you. It destroys what you're *not*.

The burning is not the breakdown. It's the refining. And you don't have to torch your whole life. You just have to stop protecting the parts that are already ashes.

What Are You Still Carrying That's Not Yours?

So much of what weighs us down isn't even ours. It's inherited expectation. Outdated ambition. Roles we never meant to keep. Beliefs we absorbed without questioning.

We carry:

- The version of success someone else handed us
- The identity we once needed to survive — but no longer do
- The pressure to be strong, capable, calm, brilliant, all the time

- The rhythm that served a past season, but drains us now.

We carry things long after they've expired — out of loyalty, fear, or simple momentum.

And at some point, it becomes too heavy. Not because you're weak. But because you were never meant to carry all of this in the first place. You are allowed to set it down. You don't have to explain. You don't need a dramatic exit. You just need to be honest enough to say: *"This no longer fits."* You're not failing. You're shedding.

And what you let go of now?

That's what makes space for who you're becoming.

Death of a Former Self

Let's name it clearly:

Reinvention requires a death.

Not a gentle rebrand. Not a tidy upgrade. A letting go so full and final it feels like loss — because it is. The version of you that people knew, that *you* knew — is gone. And that's not a bad thing. But it is something to honour.

It might be:

- The career you gave your best years to
- The identity that made you feel powerful — or safe
- The dream that once lit you up, but no longer does
- The part of you that kept everyone else comfortable

Letting her go can feel like betrayal. But clinging to her becomes its own kind of self-abandonment. You can't become who you're here to be while dragging who you used to be behind you.

There is grief in this.

Even when it's the right choice. Even when you're ready. Even when the new you is brighter, calmer, more whole — you'll still miss parts of the old.

That's OK. You can hold reverence for who you were…while choosing not to keep performing her.

This isn't a collapse. It's a shedding. A rite of passage. A necessary death, so something more true can live.

Resistance to the Burn

Even when you know it's time — you might resist the fire. You might light the match… and blow it out. You might walk toward the edge… and talk yourself back into the same old rhythm. You might say, *"Soon."* And keep saying it for years. This is normal.

We resist for good reasons.

Because letting go means letting people down. It means becoming someone others didn't expect. It means releasing an identity that once made you proud — even if now it just makes you tired.

Here's what resistance often sounds like:

- *"What if I regret this?"*
- *"What will people think?"*
- *"I can't just stop now."*
- *"This is who I am."*
- *"But I've already come so far."*

And yet… your soul keeps whispering: *"You've already outgrown this."*

There's no such thing as a tidy burn. Trying to keep one hand on the old while reaching for the new? It stretches you thin. Keeps you stuck in-between. Exhausts you. You don't need to leap.

But you do need to choose.

Letting go doesn't mean setting fire to everything. But it does mean being honest about what's already smouldering — and letting it go completely, instead of pretending it's still alive.

What Survives the Fire

Here's the most surprising part of letting the old burn:

You don't lose everything.

In fact, what survives the fire is the most true, the most durable, the most *you*. After the old roles, rhythms, and rules are gone... what remains?

- Your voice
- Your values
- Your grit
- Your intuition
- Your sense of humour
- Your ability to rebuild — this time, with intention

Letting go doesn't erase who you are. It reveals it. Because so much of what you thought defined you — the job title, the awards, the reputation, the pace — was never the core. It was the armour. The costume. The casing.

What burns away is what you *aren't*.

What's left is what you *are*.

After cancer treatment, it was like I'd been through the fire. No hair. Fewer brain cells. No strength. No glow. I wasn't myself — or at least, not the version I had recognised for years.

I was down to nothing. No — not nothing. I was down to the

core. Like a mass of rock that had been broken, sifted, burned — until only one solitary gem remained. The essence of me.

What surprised me most was realising that this quiet, stripped-back version... was still me. The strength had changed. The clarity had deepened. And the noise had finally fallen away. I wasn't lost.

I was refined.

* * *

You don't have to fear the fire. It's not coming to destroy you. It's coming to clarify you. And in that clarity, something extraordinary happens. You begin again — not from scratch, but from truth.

The Bravery of Letting Go Publicly

It's one thing to burn the old in private. To make a quiet decision in your heart. To whisper to yourself, *"I'm done."*

But it's another thing entirely to let go... *where people can see you*. To stop performing the role everyone recognises. To step away from the thing they admired you for. To change direction when everyone thought you were thriving.

And suddenly, the questions begin:

- *"Why would you give that up?"*
- *"Are you sure?"*
- *"What are you doing next?"*
- *"Are you OK?"*

They mean well. But their discomfort can make you doubt your clarity.

Letting go is brave.

But *letting go publicly* — that's a new level of courage. Because not only are you releasing something familiar — you're doing it without a tidy script, while being watched.

But here's the truth:

You don't need everyone to understand.

You don't need a perfect answer.

You don't need to make it look polished or explain it on Instagram.

You just need to honour the quiet, inconvenient, powerful truth: *"This is no longer mine to carry."* Because every time you do that — every time you burn something outdated and stand tall in the smoke — you give others permission to do the same.

The Controlled Burn

In forest management, there's a technique called the *controlled burn*. It's not reckless destruction. It's not failure. It's an intentional fire — deliberately set to clear out what's dead, overgrown, or invasive.

Why?

Because without it, the forest becomes too dense. The old brush suffocates the soil. New growth can't break through. So the rangers set fire to it — on purpose. They don't panic. They plan. They create space. They let the fire do what it's meant to do.

And when it's over? What's left is soil that's richer. Roots that are stronger. And space — glorious space — for life to begin again. This is what letting go can be. You don't have to torch your whole life.

You just have to stop clinging to what's already dying. You get to be the one who says: *"This part is no longer healthy. It's time to clear it."*

Not because you're in crisis. But because you're wise enough to make room for what's next.

The fire isn't the end. It's the beginning of growth you can't yet see.

A Wise Woman's Words

"Maybe for me, all those years ago, one moment when I said no more was when I asked my husband to leave the house and said no to more abuse from him for me or my daughters.

I had a high school education, no skills, no money, no way to support myself or my children, had never worked outside the home, no social system to catch me, no family to go back to—and 4 toddlers still clinging to my skirts.

I got a job in a donut shop, paying $1 an hour and we literally survived on stale donuts for several weeks which I took home at the end of the night.

My kids loved it!

And now, here I am - living in a stunningly beautiful place, a relationship beyond my wildest imagination, talking to beautiful, fascinating people.

Who would have thought it?"

— Jeannie

Reflection — What's Already Ashes?

Take a breath. Be honest. Be kind to the version of you that kept going, even when the flame had already gone out. Some things are over before we admit they're over. Not because we're weak — but because we're loyal. To the version of us that once needed it. To the story we hoped would last. To the role we built a whole life around.

But pretending something's still on fire doesn't make it burn again. It just leaves you standing in smoke.

Journal Moment

- What part of your life feels heavy, hollow, or forced — even if it still looks fine from the outside?
- What identity are you still performing out of habit or history — but no longer feel connected to?
- What would you gently release if you didn't need anyone's approval to let it go?
- What truth are you avoiding because it would mean letting go of something that once defined you?

Letting go is brave. But sometimes, just *admitting* what's already gone is the most powerful act of all.

Pause. Reflect. Realign.

There is something new ready to rise — but first, give yourself permission to stop pretending.

Edge Move — Burn One Thing

This week, choose one thing to release. A commitment. A title. A role. A rhythm. A belief that no longer fits.

Write it down. Say it aloud. Burn it — if you can safely do so — or tear it, shred it, bury it.

Then say: *"I release what no longer fits. I trust what remains."*

This is not destruction. This is renewal. You are not becoming less. You are becoming *true*.

Part Three
Walking Forward, Your Way

Chapter 11
Reclaiming Joy

The Space Joy Walks Into

Joy doesn't show up with a drumroll. It arrives quietly, in the space you never used to leave. It walks in through the door that burnout blew open. Not when you're chasing it. Not when you're braced for it. But when you've finally made enough space — not just in your schedule, but in yourself.

For me, joy didn't return in some grand, life-changing moment. It came back in fragments. A song I forgot I loved. Laughter with a friend that felt easy again. A walk without headphones. A deep breath that didn't feel rushed.

It didn't feel productive. It didn't look impressive. But it felt like life again.

* * *

I was queuing at the airport to fly to Germany. It had been a long day — the usual shuffle of passports, baggage, and body scans. I had my headphones in, half tuned out, half lost in a beat. Franc

Moody was playing — a favourite of mine — and without meaning to, I started moving...

Nothing dramatic. Just a small bounce, a shoulder roll, a rhythm in my step.

The guy behind me smiled.

That's when I realised I was grinning. Fully grinning. Not for anyone. Not for a camera. Just... because.

It caught me off guard — this joy that snuck up on me, not staged or structured. I wasn't trying to impress anyone. I wasn't rushing to be anywhere else. For that one minute, I was simply myself. Unedited. Undone in the best possible way.

That's when you know something in you has shifted. When joy stops needing permission. When it returns not with fanfare, but with headphones, a beat, and a queue at gate 46.

* * *

For a long time, I thought joy was something I had to earn. After the work. After the goals. After I'd proved I was useful enough, strong enough, successful enough. But joy doesn't wait at the finish line. It lives in the pause. The moment after the letting go. The breath that says, *"You made it."* You don't chase it.

You clear space — and let it walk in.

The Difference Between Performing Happiness and Feeling Joy

We live in a world where happiness performs well. It photographs well. It captions well. Smiles for the camera. Gratitude lists. "So lucky, so grateful." And maybe it's all true.

But sometimes — it's also a script. We learn early how to *look* joyful. To tick the boxes, say the right things, keep the energy up. Especially if we're leaders, business owners, caregivers — we know how to beam, reassure, and "bring the vibe." But that's not joy. That's *performance*.

Real joy is quieter.

It doesn't need to prove anything. It doesn't need an audience. You can be joyful alone on a Tuesday, in your kitchen, singing to a song no one else hears. You can feel it on a walk with no phone, when your shoulders drop and something in you says, *"This is it."*

Joy doesn't always look happy. Sometimes it looks like calm. Sometimes it looks like presence. Sometimes it looks like choosing not to go to the party — and feeling completely OK about that.

The difference isn't always obvious on the outside. But inside? It's everything. One leaves you drained. The other fills you, quietly, without needing applause.

What Stole It in the First Place

Joy rarely disappears all at once. It's not a dramatic exit. It slips away quietly, over time — beneath the weight of everything else. So what steals it?

Often, it's not trauma or crisis. It's pace. Pressure. Pretence. It's living in overdrive, managing too much, and pausing too little.

Here are some of the most common joy-thieves:

- **Over-functioning.** You do everything for everyone. Competent? Yes. Joyful? Not really.
- **Over-achieving.** You chase success, tick boxes, hit goals — and still feel oddly empty.
- **People-pleasing.** You smile. Say yes. Show up. Perform. Then collapse in private.
- **Productivity addiction.** You earn rest like it's a luxury — not a necessity.
- **Chronic self-editing.** You filter yourself. You

shrink. You manage other people's comfort instead of honouring your own clarity.
- **Postponed joy.** You put off fun until everything's done. Spoiler: it's never all done.

Sound familiar?

* * *

I remember sitting with a dear friend of mine, Val, one of those rare people who was equal parts counsellor, cheerleader, and truth-teller.

At the time, I was deep in the thick of it: running two businesses, raising three little ones, juggling all the plates with that familiar tight smile. We were catching up over coffee, and I gave her the usual update — things were going well, business was thriving, awards were rolling in. All the external markers looked shiny.

She listened quietly, then looked me straight in the eye and asked:

"But what are you doing for fun?"

I opened my mouth to answer — and nothing came out. I couldn't think of a single thing. Not one.

In all the noise and doing and proving, joy had quietly slipped out the back door. And I hadn't even noticed it was gone.

* * *

Joy doesn't need a reason to exist. But it *does* need room. And the moment you start clearing out what stole it — it starts making its way back.

You Don't Have to Earn Joy

Let's just say it:

You don't have to earn your joy. Not by finishing your to-do list. Not by being good, or useful, or impressive. Not by holding it all together. Not by proving how much you've suffered. Joy is not a reward for enduring enough pain. It's not a badge you get after surviving.

It's your birthright. Your blueprint. It's in you.

And yet — how often do we postpone it?

- *I'll rest when the launch is done.*
- *I'll celebrate when it's perfect.*
- *I'll have fun when things settle down.*

But what if things never settle down? What if joy is the thing that would *carry you* through the mess — not wait patiently on the other side of it?

* * *

There was a moment during chemo. Everything in my body was tired — the kind of tired that doesn't lift with rest. My world had narrowed to small things: medication schedules, side effects, energy conservation. But one day, I took a short walk. Just a few minutes outside.

I looked up. The sky was a soft, open blue. A bird sang — high and light, unaware of everything. And there it was.

Joy.

Not loud. Not manic. Just a flicker of peace that landed in my chest and stayed there, warming me from the inside out. That one moment gave me strength. It reminded me that joy isn't something you earn after the hard part is over — it's something that *can* walk beside you, even in the middle of it all.

You don't have to feel guilty for feeling good. You don't have to apologise for being lit up when others are heavy. You don't have to tone it down to be taken seriously. Let joy live here, now, in the middle.

Not as the prize — but as the *power source.*

Small Joy Is Real Joy

Not all joy is life-changing. Sometimes it's life-*sustaining.* We're conditioned to chase the big moments. The launch. The trip. The milestone.

But the most nourishing joy? It often arrives quietly — in the in-between. Tiny moments. Simple sparks. Un-instagrammable bliss. Real joy isn't always dramatic. It's subtle. Slow. Sneaky.

Small joy may look like:

- Sunlight pouring across the kitchen floor
- A deep exhale when you cancel something you didn't want to do
- Singing in the car — loud, off-key, windows down
- A message from someone who just *gets* you
- Laughing until your stomach hurts
- The first sip of coffee before anyone else wakes up
- That feeling after moving your body — not to punish it, but to return to it
- Catching your reflection and thinking, *"I like her."*
- Saying no — and not feeling guilty
- Saying yes — to yourself.

Have you ever looked in the mirror — not at your hair, not at your makeup — but into your eyes? One day, I did. I paused. I really looked. And for a moment, something shifted. I caught myself looking back. It was strange. And strangely beautiful.

We smiled at each other.

I liked her. She looked fun. She looked like she had joy. I wanted to spend more time with her. That was the moment I realised — I didn't want to "get back to normal." Not back to who I used to be. The new, refined version of me was right there.

And this time, I saw her.

These moments don't need an audience. They don't need to be shared. They just need to be noticed — and felt. Because the more you honour them? The more they multiply.

Joy After Pain Feels Different

There's a kind of joy you earn — not through achievement, but through endurance. It's not the giddy, fizzy kind you felt at fourteen. It's slower. Deeper. Heavier in the best way. Joy after pain is different.

It arrives without fanfare. It doesn't demand anything. It simply sits beside you like an old friend, quietly saying:

"You're still here."

And somehow, that's enough. This is joy that's been through something. Joy that knows grief. Joy that didn't think it would return — and did.

* * *

When I was diagnosed, the cancer was advanced— stage 4, it obviously wasn't ideal. The first round of chemo broke the lymphoma down so quickly that it almost broke me too. One night, I was shaking uncontrollably. I think an ambulance took me to Emergency — but honestly, I can't really remember. It's all a blur.

What I *do* remember is this.

In the middle of that moment — not knowing if I'd make it through the night — I looked at my loved ones... and I didn't feel fear. I felt love. And I felt deep joy. That whole period. It doesn't sit in my memory as a dark chapter. It was stripped back, yes. Raw. Painful. But underneath it all, there was more depth than I had ever felt. There was this joy.

When I was learning business, I used to read every story I could get my hands on. I wanted to learn the hard lessons without having to live every hard moment. That's how I feel about what illness taught me. I wish I could hand over the knowing, without anyone needing to live through the pain. But it's hard to articulate — hard to pin down in a single sentence.

What I learned was this:

Life is short. And most of what we stress over doesn't matter. But oddly, what I longed for most during those months wasn't big bucket-list adventures.

It was the ordinary.

I wanted to walk to the shop. To make tea. To smile. To just *be*. Not to "live like every day is your last" — but to have the *luxury* of forgetting that it might be.

That, to me, is joy.

Not the kind you post on Instagram. Not the holiday or the headline kind. But something deeper. The kind of joy that holds you when everything else falls away.

Joy after pain doesn't erase the past. It coexists with it. It makes space for everything that came before — and says, *"You can feel this too."* It doesn't mean everything's perfect. It just means something is possible again.

Joy that returns after the fire is not naive.

It's sacred. And the fact that you can feel it again — even just for a moment — means something is healing.

Let Joy Be the Compass Now

We're taught to make decisions based on logic, duty, responsibility, or 'return on investment.' But what if we let joy lead? Not recklessness. Not avoidance. But honest, aligned, *this-lights-me-up* joy.

What if joy wasn't the afterthought... but the compass?

Let's play:

- What if you said yes to the work that energised you — not just the work that impressed people?
- What if you planned your diary around what made you feel alive — not just what made you feel accomplished?
- What if you said no to the things that drain you — even if they're "good" things?
- What if ease didn't mean lazy?
- What if fun *counted*?
- What if joy wasn't a break from real life... but the *point* of it?

Here's what I know. When I let joy steer — I don't drift. I don't lose focus. I become *clearer*. Because joy clarifies what matters. It lifts the fog.

Have you ever had a cold shower? Sometimes, I wake up with my mind in a blur — foggy, heavy, dulled by sleep. I ease myself into the shower slowly, bracing. And then it hits — the rush of cold water on my skin. Suddenly, I'm *here*. Present. Awake. Clear. Every cell alive again.

That's what joy does. It doesn't just comfort — it *cuts through*.

It wakes you up. Reminds you who you are. And in that split second, everything that doesn't matter… just falls away.

It shows you the difference between what you *can* do and what you *want* to do. And when you follow it — even a little — life gets louder in colour.

The Wildflower Return

After a forest fire, something surprising happens. The first things to grow back aren't the tallest trees or the strongest roots. They're wildflowers. Tiny. Bright. Unexpected. They arrive not in spite of the burn — but *because of it.*

The fire clears the space. And in that space, seeds that had been buried — dormant for years — finally get light. They bloom.

Joy is like that.

It doesn't always return how you expect. Not through a grand event or a life-changing epiphany. Sometimes it returns in colour, in softness, in something small you almost missed. It grows in the cracks. In the spaces you once thought were ruined. In the middle of your new, uncertain, spacious life.

And one day, you look around — and realise. You didn't lose yourself. You made room for yourself. And joy came back, wild and free, because it could finally breathe again.

Reflection — Where Is Joy Waiting for You?

Let this be a moment to tune in. Not to achieve. Not to prove. Just to *notice.*

Joy doesn't demand much. It doesn't schedule itself in your diary. It doesn't need you to earn it first. It just needs you to stop long enough to feel it. It can arrive in a breath. In the first sip of coffee. In a laugh that takes you by surprise. In the light across your kitchen floor.

Journal Moment

- What kind of joy feels most true to you right now — gentle, playful, wild, still?
- Where have you been performing happiness — and where have you actually *felt* it?
- What small moment in the past week lifted you more than you expected?
- What did you once love that still lives in you, waiting to be welcomed back?

You don't have to fix your whole life to feel joy. You don't have to escape to find it. You just have to stop rushing past it. Because joy isn't loud. It waits in quiet corners. It rises when you let yourself *be* — without armour, without agenda.

Pause. Reflect. Realign.

Joy is a quiet kind of knowing. It doesn't chase — and it can't be chased. It arrives when you become still enough to notice… and soft enough to let it in.

Edge Move — Schedule Joy

This week, don't wait for joy to "fit in." Make space for it — on purpose. Even if it's small. Especially if it's small. Pick something that feels good for *no reason*. Something that doesn't earn you points, followers, praise, or income. Something that delights you. Calms you. Returns you to yourself.

- A walk with no destination
- Your favourite song — on repeat

- A bath with no podcast, no agenda
- A café trip alone with a good book
- Dancing in your kitchen
- Saying no, and then exhaling

And here's the most important part:

Don't explain it. Don't justify it. Don't multitask while doing it.

Just let joy be *the point*.

Write it into your diary like a meeting that matters — because it does. Joy doesn't need a reason.

It just needs room.

Chapter 12
Becoming You Again

"I don't care what you think about me. I don't think about you at all."

— Coco Chanel

The Moment You Realise You're Not Lost

You weren't broken. You didn't disappear. You didn't fail. You just drifted.

Bit by bit, under the weight of what life asked of you — the roles, the rhythm, the rush — you forgot how to hear your own voice. But one day... something shifts. It's not loud. It's not dramatic. It's often ridiculously simple.

A moment of stillness. A laugh that comes from somewhere deeper. A spark of energy when you speak the truth — and don't filter it.

For me, it wasn't a grand transformation. It was a moment in the mountains, or laughing uncontrollably with someone who really sees me, or standing still and breathing — and feeling fully, *finally*, like myself again.

* * *

I love chatting to strangers. It happens all the time in the mountains. You pass someone on the path and it starts with a smile. Then a "Hi." Then, somehow, "How's your day been?" Before you know it, you're swapping stories. Where have you come from? Where are you going? And just like that — a laugh, a spark, a little exchange of joy.

No phones. No small talk. Just two people, briefly human together, somewhere between a summit and a descent. Those are the moments I feel most myself.

Unrushed. Unperformed. Just present. And every time, a quiet thought rises up:

There I am.

* * *

It's not a reinvention. It's a return. You look around and realise:

You've been under the surface all along — just waiting for the noise to quiet so you could rise again.

You don't need to start over. You just need to *uncover* the parts of you that still remember who you are.

Unbecoming Isn't Regressing

Here's the myth:

If you start letting go — of the roles, the rhythm, the relentless pace — you're somehow *going backwards.*

You're not.

You're unbecoming everything you never meant to carry. You're unclenching. Uncrowding. Unfiltering. You're not shrinking — you're shedding.

This isn't regression. It's refinement.

You're returning to a version of yourself who was always there — under the ambition, under the calendar, under the "I've got this" smile. Not the you from ten years ago.

The *real* you. The un-edited, fully-alive version that doesn't need to perform strength to be strong.

Unbecoming isn't weak. It's wildly intelligent. Because once you stop performing for the room, you get to actually feel like yourself *in* the room. And it turns out — she's a lot more powerful than the version you were trying to be.

All the Roles You Tried On

At some point, we all pick up a few extra identities — just to get by, get ahead, or keep the peace. We try on roles like outfits, hoping one will make us feel settled. And they work... for a while.

Maybe you became:

- The Achiever — always saying yes, always exceeding expectations
- The Fixer — solving everyone's problems, even the ones they didn't ask you to fix
- The Expert — needing to have the answers, especially when you're secretly exhausted
- The Pleaser — softening your edges to stay agreeable
- The Calm One — performing peace while screaming internally
- The Reliable One — forgetting what you want because you're managing what everyone else needs

I used to carry a lot of labels. Mother. Sister. Daughter. Friend. Employer. Principal. Businesswoman. Dentist. Charity chair. Editor. Survivor. Facilitator. Women's rights advocate. Leader.

Each one came with a script. A certain polish. A sense of duty.

And somewhere along the way, without realising it, I had started performing them — instead of simply *being*.

When I became ill, one of the first roles to shift was that of "all-knowing mother." I couldn't be the caregiver anymore. The chemo brought memory loss and confusion — and suddenly, my children became the ones gently supporting me. We met each other as humans. The hierarchy fell away. And in its place: something more honest. Something equal. Something better.

That shift changed everything.

It flowed into my other roles, too — as a leader, a colleague, a woman. I no longer need to be the expert. I just want to be in the room.

None of these roles were bad. They helped me survive, succeed, stay safe. They served a purpose. But the thing about roles? They're not your whole story. They're scripts — and at some point, you outgrow the lines. You wake up one day and think:

"This isn't me anymore. It never fully was."

That's not failure. That's freedom. It's not about throwing everything out — it's about deciding what's *actually yours*, and what you were just holding because it made other people comfortable.

Signs You've Drifted from Yourself

Sometimes, you don't realise how far you've drifted until you feel slightly... off. Not broken. Not burnt out. Just not *quite* you.

Here are a few clues:

- You stare at a menu and don't know what you like anymore.
- You keep saying "I'm fine" — and almost believe it.
- You feel weirdly tired after being around people who used to energise you.

- You can't remember the last time you belly-laughed — or said exactly what you meant.
- You edit your words mid-sentence to avoid discomfort.
- You keep thinking, *"I'll feel more like myself when…"* — but that moment never quite comes.

Drift doesn't happen all at once. It's subtle. It's cumulative. It's small compromises stacked on top of each other until you look up and think, *"Wait — where did I go?"* The good news? You're still there. You don't have to blow up your life to return.

You just have to start listening for the moments that feel like *you* — and follow them.

Glimmers of the Real You Returning

Coming back to yourself isn't a big reveal. It's more like… remembering. Flashes. Glimmers. Quiet "oh, there I am" moments. Sometimes it happens mid-laugh, when you surprise yourself. Sometimes it's singing loudly in the car, or walking faster because you feel good. Sometimes it's not holding back in a conversation — and realising you didn't shrink.

You might:

- Wear something bold and *not* tone it down
- Say no without overexplaining
- Feel joy doing something completely ordinary
- Catch yourself smiling alone — and not immediately wiping it off

These aren't massive moves. They're signals. You're not rebuilding from scratch. You're dusting off something real. And the more you notice these glimmers, the more they grow. You don't need to hustle your way back to yourself. You just need to stop dismissing the parts that already feel right.

Reclaiming Without Apology

There's a version of you returning now — bolder, calmer, more grounded, maybe even a little louder — and she might not fit neatly into the roles you used to play.

That's OK.

You're not here to stay consistent for the comfort of others. You're here to be *real*. You might find yourself:

- Talking differently — clearer, more direct, less sugar-coated
- Dressing differently — not to impress, but to feel good
- Showing up with less small talk and more truth
- Taking up space, not filling it with apologies
- Laughing louder. Needing less permission.

Reclaiming yourself can rattle people. Not because you're too much — but because you're finally not trying to be less. And when people say:

"You've changed…"

Let your answer be:

"I've come back."

No apology. No long explanation. Just presence. Because you don't owe the world your predictability. You owe yourself your wholeness.

You know what I've realised? People are scared of honesty. I used to be scared of being honest too — always wondering, *"What will they think?"* But the truth is, honesty unsettles people. It's disarming. It interrupts the performance.

When you say what you really think — calmly, clearly, without aggression — it shifts the energy in the room. Not everyone will know how to meet that. But that doesn't mean you should soften it.

Change is inconvenient. Not just for you — but for the people around you. When you start to shift, people get uncomfortable. They liked the predictable version of you. The helpful, agreeable one. And sometimes, they'll pressure you to return to that version. Not out of cruelty — but because *your change makes them question their own comfort.*

And that's OK. You don't need to be digestible. You just need to be *true*.

The Flavour of Change

I've always wondered how some people can just *know* what they like. "I like strawberry ice cream," they say, with conviction. And I think — *how do you know?*

Because honestly, I don't always know what I like.

Chocolate? Vanilla? Depends on the day. What kind of mood am I in? What have I just eaten? Yesterday I liked chocolate. Today, I'm not even sure I like ice cream at all — especially not with all that high-GI refined sugar. Today, I'd rather have a coffee.

That's the thing — we change.

Our tastes change. Our thinking changes. Who I am today isn't quite who I was yesterday. And I'm already shifting into who I'll be tomorrow. The life that fit me then? It doesn't fit anymore. And when that happens — it's not a crisis.

It's a cue. It means I need to change. To realign. To stop trying to force myself back into the flavour I've outgrown.

The Undo Button

Becoming yourself again doesn't feel like a makeover. It feels like hitting "undo" on a document you over-edited. You started with something solid. Something true.

Then life handed you red pens:

- *Be more professional here.*
- *Tone that bit down.*
- *Add something more agreeable.*
- *Delete that — it's too much.*
- *Let's swap clarity for likability.*

You didn't mean to lose yourself. You were just trying to make the story better. Safer. More acceptable. But somewhere in all the edits, the essence got lost. And now? You're finding the undo button.

Each time you laugh louder. Say no faster. Tell the truth more clearly — you undo another layer of someone else's script.

And what's left?

You.

The original draft. Full of energy, colour, opinion, edge. Less polished — but infinitely more powerful. Turns out, she didn't need rewriting. She just needed reclaiming.

Voice from the Edge

"My husband had an incredible job offer in America—too good to ignore. At the time, I was working in my sweet spot, finally reaping the rewards of years of hard graft getting my bachelor's and master's degrees. It was a no-brainer to give him the world.

What I hadn't accounted for was this: I hate change. I love my family (as nuts as they are). And I loved Scotland—my chosen country, my home.

As he thrived, my heart slowly broke—being away from everything and everyone I loved, day after day.

I had a choice: leave and go home, stay stuck in misery, or embrace this new norm.

It took time, but I chose the latter.

To my surprise, dear friends became my family away from home. After trying several jobs—some I loved, others I hated—I started to remember who I was. The smart, funny, kind girl I'd always been.

I made it my business to shine, wherever I was.

It didn't happen overnight, but I worked hard, persevered, and found a role where I use all my gifts and talents—and I'm appreciated for who I am.

Success was redefined for me.

Don't ever give up—joy comes in the morning.

Be confident in who you are.

Break the mold.

Be unapologetically you."

— My Friend from her edge.

Reflection — Who Are You Without the Edits?

Pause.

Breathe.

Check in — not with the version of you the world sees, but with the one quietly waiting underneath.

The one who existed before the roles.

Before the titles.

Before the carefully curated, slightly-too-polished version of a self you've outgrown.

That person? She's still there.

Maybe a little quieter now.

Maybe hidden under a few layers of shoulds.

But never gone.

Journal Moment

- What part of you have you missed — and what might it need to come back?
- What identity are you still wearing because it makes others more comfortable?
- Where are you most yourself — a time of day, a place, a relationship, a silence?
- What do you keep saying yes to — that your spirit has already said no to?
- What would it feel like to stop editing — and show up just as you are?

You're not lost. You've just learned to perform a version of yourself that helped you survive.

And now, you're safe enough to come home.

Pause. Reflect. Realign.

You don't have to reinvent yourself.
 You just have to remove what was never really you.
 And when you do — you'll find you were there all along.
 Still whole. Still worthy. Still waiting.

Edge Move — Do Something Unedited

This week, give yourself one moment of full, unapologetic *you*. Something unedited. Unfiltered. Slightly louder or softer or sillier than usual.

Maybe it's:

Lead from the Edge

- Saying what you really think — kindly, clearly
- Wearing what makes you feel alive — not just appropriate
- Taking up space in a room, without shrinking or smoothing
- Turning down a plan you don't want, without a 200-word excuse
- Singing. Dancing. Playing. Anything that says, *"I'm back."*

You don't owe anyone the quiet version of you. You don't need permission to return.

You were always there — just waiting to be heard.

Chapter 13
Strength That Doesn't Shout

> "It took me quite a long time to develop a voice, and now that I have it, I am not going to be silent."
> —*Madeleine Albright*

Redefining what power looks and feels like

There's a kind of power that doesn't announce itself. It doesn't interrupt, dominate, or overcompensate. It doesn't need a platform, a spotlight, or a microphone. It simply is — steady, grounded, quiet in its confidence. Real strength doesn't need to prove itself. It holds the room without raising its voice.

The Old Script of Strength

For years, I thought power meant being the loudest. The one who always knew the answer. The one who walked into the room with energy turned up to eleven and made things happen, fast.

In many ways, that version of me worked — she built businesses, made waves, got things done. But underneath all that volume was an edge I didn't yet understand: I was driving, not leading. Pushing, not guiding. And I was tired.

Discovering a New Kind of Power

When life brought me to the edge — illness, identity shifts, a stripping away of what no longer served — I discovered something I hadn't seen before: quiet strength.

The kind that listens more than it speaks. That holds space instead of filling it. That trusts, rather than controls. It wasn't weakness. It was deeper, more spacious, and far more enduring.

The Myth That Softness Is Weakness

This chapter is an invitation to redefine what strength looks like, especially if you've been taught that leadership requires noise, certainty, or performance. It's for the ones who've been told they're "too soft" or "not forceful enough" — and for those, like I once was, who fear that softening means shrinking.

Here, we explore how strength lives in stillness, in boundaries, in resilience that doesn't need applause. We'll talk about holding your centre when things wobble, finding your voice without shouting,

and walking into rooms — or out of them — with the quiet confidence of someone who no longer needs to prove a thing.

The Anatomy of Quiet Strength

Most of us have been taught that strength is something you show — something external. But quiet strength is an inner stance, not an outward performance.

It's a way of being that creates impact without volume.

Here are five core elements of quiet strength that redefine how we lead, connect, and stand in our power:

1. Presence Over Performance

True strength starts with presence — the ability to be fully here, fully yourself, without needing to convince, entertain, or impress.

It's not what you say that carries power; it's the energy you bring when you walk into a room. People feel presence. They lean toward it. It invites trust.

2. Clarity Over Control

Control feels powerful in the short term, but it's rooted in fear. Quiet strength trusts clarity instead — a grounded knowing of your values, direction, and boundaries.

From that place, you don't need to micromanage or manipulate outcomes. You lead with intention, not anxiety.

3. Boundaries Over Busyness

There's a quiet kind of power in saying no — in choosing wisely where your time, energy, and presence go. Over-giving, overworking, and overcommitting are often mistaken for dedication,

but they're usually signs we've lost connection to our centre. Quiet strength honours limits as an act of leadership.

4. Listening Over Speaking

In a world of noise, listening is radical. It's powerful to be the person who waits, who pays attention, who creates space for others to be heard.

Quiet strength listens — not just with ears, but with curiosity, empathy, and intuition. It allows for depth over dominance.

5. Stillness Over Speed

Quiet strength knows when to act — and when to wait. It's not passive, but it isn't frantic. It doesn't rush toward solutions to avoid discomfort.

It can sit with the unknown. It has patience. It knows that not everything powerful needs to be fast.

This version of strength may not be loud — but it's immovable. It doesn't need a megaphone to be felt. It doesn't need applause to be valid.

It's the kind of power that stays when the performance ends, when the crisis passes, and when the next chapter begins.

* * *

I was in a strategy meeting. Everyone had weighed in — my team, the consultant, the energy in the room pushing toward a unanimous decision. I listened. I considered. And then, quietly, I said, "I disagree."

The room was still.

That was quiet strength. Not defiance. Not performance. Just rooted clarity.

Just because the majority agrees doesn't mean your voice doesn't belong. You don't need to shout to be heard. You just need to trust your ground.

Strength in Stillness

There were times during illness when I couldn't lead, couldn't talk, couldn't plan. But I could still hold presence. Stillness became its own form of power — not passive, but deeply aware. There's something quietly formidable about someone who can stay present in discomfort without rushing to fix it.

Voice from the Edge

— A story shared by a dear colleague and friend

Lead from the Edge

I just wanted to share...

My edges have been sharp.

From a challenging childhood — the eldest of four — I grew up fast. My mum struggled with schizophrenia from the time I was six. She was either in hospital, in bed, or so heavily medicated that daily life at home fell to me. I cooked, did laundry, and managed the house. That was just how it was.

By the age of ten, I had decided I wanted to be a dentist. I liked the uniform.

All through GCSEs and A-levels, my responsibilities at home didn't stop. And while I never questioned whether I'd keep going, the system often questioned me.

I still remember the words of my deputy headmaster when I said I wanted to study dentistry:

"I don't think you're clever enough."

Those words stuck. Especially on A-level results day.

I went to school, opened the envelope — and saw I hadn't achieved the grades I needed to get into Newcastle University, my first choice. I was devastated. Inconsolable.

And then — the same deputy head said:

"Just give the admissions tutor a call."

Through floods of tears, I did. And somehow, they let me in anyway.

Looking back now, I see it wasn't just about getting into university.

It was about believing in myself, even when others didn't.

Five years of dental school followed. In my first year, I failed anatomy by just 1%. Anxiety got the better of me in the viva. But I picked myself up and sat it again — second time around, I scored 96%. I haven't looked back since.

This year marks 27 years since I qualified. I've owned a dental practice, have a special interest in endodontics, worked for UK Sedation, and founded my own aesthetics studio.

And through it all, I've learned this:
Resilience isn't about never breaking. It's about returning again and again.
— Laura Carr

Reflection — Where Does Your Strength Live?

Not all strength is loud. Not all power is visible. Some of the deepest strength shows up when no one's watching. When there's no applause. No performance. No pressure.

Just you — showing up anyway.

This reflection is for the strength you might overlook… because it doesn't look like the kind the world rewards.

Journal Moment

- When do you feel most grounded, centred, or quietly powerful — even if no one else notices?
- What habits or patterns lead you to overperform, overprove, or overcompensate?
- Where are you acting strong… but feeling stretched thin beneath the surface?
- Who in your life models quiet strength — and what do they teach you about how presence can hold more power than performance?
- What might shift if you stopped trying to be impressive — and chose to be *true* instead?

You don't have to prove your strength to anyone. Sometimes, it's the soft stance.

The stillness.

The silent "no" or the calm "I disagree" that carries the most impact.

Pause. Reflect. Realign.

Strength doesn't have to announce itself.

It can whisper.

It can breathe.

It can simply hold its ground and choose not to shrink.

Let yourself redefine what powerful really feels like — when it comes from within.

Edge Move: The Quiet Centre

This is a short, grounding practice you can do anytime you feel the urge to rush, prove, or push.

1. Stop what you're doing. Sit or stand still. Let your body settle — not into collapse, but into steadiness.
2. Feel your feet. Place both feet flat on the ground. Imagine strength rising up from the earth through your heels.
3. Take three slow breaths. In through the nose. Out through the mouth. Each breath, let a little more tension drop away.
4. Drop in and ask: "What would strength look like if I didn't have to prove it?"
5. Wait. Listen. Don't force an answer. Just notice what rises. A word. A feeling. A gesture. Trust that your body knows

This version of strength may not be loud — but it's immovable. It doesn't need a megaphone to be felt. It doesn't need applause to be valid. It stays after the performance ends. It stays through the wobble. It stays when the next chapter begins.

And so do you.

Chapter 14
Trusting the Process

"The process is the point."

When You Want a Straight Line — and Life Gives You Spirals

Wouldn't it be nice if growth came with a map? A neat little route from stuck → breakthrough → glow-up, with clearly marked signs and no detours.

But that's not how it goes.

Most of the time, it's more like:

- One step forward
- Two steps sideways
- Brief identity crisis
- Unplanned pivot
- Accidental breakthrough
- Sudden calm
- And repeat

Progress doesn't feel like progress when you're in it. It feels like confusion. Like waiting. Like wondering if you're doing it all wrong. We love a straight line because it gives us the illusion of control. But the spiral? The detour? The pause?

That's where the real shift happens.

You don't need to see the whole route. You just need to trust that you're not lost — just moving in a direction your future self will understand.

The Lie of Linear Progress

We love the idea that growth follows a straight line. It makes us feel in control. Logical. On track.

You do the work → you get the result.

You survive the hard thing → you bounce back.

You rest → you recover. Neatly. Predictably.

But that's not how it works. Real progress doesn't move in a straight line. It loops. Slips. Doubles back. It surprises you — sometimes with joy, often with exhaustion.

After six months of chemo and radiation therapy, I assumed recovery would be a straight line. I'd survived the hard bit. Now it was time to get better, right? So I started doing more — and instantly felt worse. Not just a little worse. Much worse. I'd take one step forward... and sink ten steps back. It felt cruel. Like I'd survived only to live in a body that couldn't keep up with life anymore.

Still, slowly — *painfully slowly* — I'd take another step. Then go back five. I'd walk around the garden... and need two weeks to recover. A few months later, I walked the same loop — and only needed one week.

That was progress.

Not the kind you post on Instagram. Not the neat graph kind.

But the slow, unpredictable, deeply human kind. I didn't know it would take five years to feel strong again.

And even now — I don't feel the *same*. I feel different.

Everything's changed. And I don't compare myself anymore. I'm not "getting back."

I'm becoming *me*.

Progress isn't a straight climb. Sometimes it's crawling. Sometimes it's sitting still and breathing. Sometimes it's a powerful pause that keeps you from burning out. Let go of the idea that you should be "further along."

You're not behind. You're in it.

Healing (and Reinvention) Take the Time They Take

We love a timeline.

"How long until I feel better?"

"How many weeks until I'm back to normal?"

"When will I stop feeling like this?"

But here's what I've learned. There is no fixed timetable for healing. Or for reinvention. Or rebuilding. Or figuring it all out. It takes the time it takes. Not because you're doing it wrong — but because you're doing it *fully*.

If someone had told me it would take five years to recover... I don't know how I would've felt. Maybe it's better I didn't know at the time. Because five years sounds like forever when you're in pain. When you're tired. When you're grieving a version of yourself that feels like it might never come back.

But if I could go back and whisper something to that version of me, it would be this:

It's worth it.

All of it — the waiting, the wondering, the inch-by-inch progress that feels invisible until one day you realise it's working.

Even if it's just for one ordinary day — where you feel calm, or strong, or joyful again — that day makes every step worth it.

Whatever your journey, hold on. You don't have to know when it ends. Just keep walking. You are not "behind." You're just moving at the speed of *real* growth. There is no deadline on becoming.

The only timeline that matters is *yours*.

* * *

I remember asking the doctors and nurses — over and over again — *"How long until I'm better?"* They were always vague. Gentle. Noncommittal. At the time, it frustrated me. I wanted answers. I wanted a date. A finish line.

I understand now.

They couldn't give me a timeline because healing doesn't follow one. Not real healing. Not the kind that changes you.

* * *

The Magic Is in the Middle

We crave the clarity of beginnings. And we celebrate the triumph of endings. But the middle? The bit between letting go and finally arriving? That part rarely gets any applause. And yet — it's where everything happens.

It's in the middle that you build resilience. It's in the middle that you question who you really are. It's in the middle that you start telling the truth — not the polished, public version, but the raw one that leads to something better.

The middle feels slow. Messy. Foggy.

Like walking through mist without knowing if the view at the top is even going to be worth it. The middle isn't glamorous. It's not inspiring in real-time.

But it's sacred.

This is where you shed what no longer fits. This is where your voice gets clearer. This is where you stop asking, *"What's the right path?"* — and start asking, *"What's the real one?"*

If you're in the middle now — don't rush it. The magic isn't waiting at the end. It's happening right here.

Trusting Yourself When You Can't See the Outcome

There's a moment — or many — where the outcome isn't clear. You've let go of what was. You haven't arrived at what's next. And no one can give you a guarantee.

This is the moment where a lot of people stall. Because we're taught to only move when we're sure. Only decide when we know it'll work. Only commit when we've run the numbers, asked the experts, and ruled out all risk. But real life doesn't give you that kind of certainty. And healing? Reinvention? Becoming?

Those are *faith-based processes.*

You don't need to have it all figured out. You don't need to see the whole map. You just need to trust yourself enough to take the next step. Then the next. Then the next.

This isn't blind hope. It's informed instinct. It's listening to your body, your breath, your clarity — even when the world is noisy.

And here's the truth:

If you only move when it's safe, you miss the moments that change you. If you wait until you're sure, you'll be waiting forever. You don't have to trust the path.

You just have to trust *yourself* to walk it.

Detaching from the Outcome Without Detaching from Yourself

Letting go of the outcome doesn't mean you stop caring. It means you stop gripping. It's the difference between planting a seed — and standing over it yelling, *"Grow faster!"* You're still showing up. Still doing the work. Still invested.

You're just no longer trying to control something that was never yours to control.

That's the edge we walk:

- Holding the vision — without holding your breath.
- Staying committed — without needing certainty.
- Trusting your path — without demanding proof.

This isn't about being passive. It's about being *present*.

You still care deeply. You still take action. You just don't tether your worth to the result. You're allowed to give your all — and then let go. And sometimes, what comes back isn't what you expected…

It's better.

* * *

The House That Moved Me

Last year, I had a quiet knowing I couldn't ignore: I needed to sell the family home.

The children had grown up and moved on. The house no longer suited my life — or the single woman I'd become. It was beautiful, full of history, and deeply familiar… but something didn't sit right anymore.

The grass always needed cutting. The repairs never stopped. I kept thinking: *This home was right for who we were. But is it right for who I am now?*

And yet — I hesitated.

I wanted my grown-up children to keep their memories. I thought maybe I should hold on to the house *for them* — even though they hadn't asked me to. So I tested the feeling. Repainted. Tidied. Tried to fall in love with it again. But no matter how polished it looked, the feeling remained: *This isn't it anymore.* I put it on the market — at a higher price than expected — and told myself: *"If I get the asking price, I'll trust it's time."*

And I did.

So I sold it. Moved into a rented place. No idea what was next. There was no plan. No dream house. No Pinterest folder. Just space.

And sometimes that's the gift — not clarity, not direction, just the absence of pressure. A pause that says: *You don't need to know yet. Just keep listening.*

I started house hunting. A smart apartment in the city — great lock-up-and-leave. A townhouse near the station — perfect for popping in and out. But I kept thinking: *Where exactly am I locking up and leaving to?*

Then, one weekend in the Lake District, I crossed a small bridge. There was a house for sale. I didn't know anyone nearby. My business wasn't there. But my heart said: *Here.*

A soft, quiet yes.

Not the life that made the most sense — but the one that made the most *peace*. This is where I want to be.

Close to the mountains. Close to the stillness.

Close to a version of myself I hadn't met yet.

Not just a house. A whole new rhythm. A whole new way of being home.

The Winding Path Up the Mountain

When you're climbing a mountain, the path doesn't go straight up. It switches back. It weaves. Sometimes it even feels like you're walking away from the summit. But every turn, every sideways step, every stretch that feels like a detour — it's all part of the ascent.

That's how process works.

You think you're not making progress because the path curves. You feel like you're stuck because the view doesn't change much between switchbacks.

But the truth is:

You're gaining elevation the whole time.

The progress is real — even when it doesn't *look* linear. You might not feel higher.

But you are.

You might not see the top yet. But you're closer than you were. You might think nothing's happening. But something is shifting — under the surface, in the soil, inside you. There's no need to rush the mountain. It's already yours.

Just keep walking.

Reflection — Where Are You Still Gripping the Outcome?

Let's take a moment to pause and turn inward. Not to figure it all out. Not to force a decision. But simply to notice where your grip is tighter than it needs to be.

Sometimes we get so fixated on the result — the clean ending, the guaranteed outcome — that we hold our breath.

We rush. We override our instincts just to make something *happen*. But growth doesn't respond to panic.

And transformation doesn't rush.

Journal Moment

- Where in your life are you demanding certainty before you move — or before you trust?
- What outcome are you gripping so tightly that it's keeping you stuck, tense, or fearful?
- Where might you loosen your hold — not to give up, but to breathe again?
- What part of your process have you been rushing, resenting, or trying to shortcut?
- What would it look like to let the process *work on you*, not just move through you?

You don't have to force your way forward. You're allowed to honour the in-between. To stay present in the pause. To walk even without the full map.

Pause. Reflect. Realign.

The process is part of the becoming.
   You don't need to know the ending to trust the path.
   Let go of gripping the outcome — and let life surprise you in ways certainty never could.

Edge Move — Walk Without the Outcome

This week, do one thing without needing a guarantee.

- Go for the walk — even if you don't know how far
- Write the thing — even if no one sees it
- Speak the truth — even if it's not perfectly received

- Let go of one deadline, one expectation, one forced timeline

And then remind yourself:
Progress doesn't have to be loud to be real. You are not behind. You are becoming — even here.
Keep walking. The path is winding. The summit is coming. And you're already on your way.

Chapter 15
The Body Remembers

When the Body Speaks Louder Than the Mind

Sometimes your body knows long before your mind admits it. "You're not stressed" — but your jaw's been locked for days. "You're not sad" — but your chest feels like it's holding something heavy. "You're fine" — but your back's screaming, your sleep's broken, and your energy is gone.

The body always tells the truth. But it speaks in sensation, not sentences. And if you're not listening — it'll find a way to get louder.

I spent years being mentally tough. Pushing through. Getting it done. And meanwhile, my body was holding the cost of all that pressure. It whispered. Then it ached. Then it shouted.

And eventually — I listened.

This chapter is about that shift. The one where we stop overriding our body's wisdom — and start respecting it. Because healing doesn't begin in your head. It begins where the pain lives. Where the tension hides.

Where your story is still being held — quietly, patiently, in the body.

What the Body Stores

You might not remember the moment — but your body does. It stores what the mind doesn't have time to process.

- The conversation where you swallowed your truth
- The email you read with a smile and a clenched jaw
- The "I'm fine" said on a day you absolutely weren't
- The grief you postponed
- The stress you normalised
- The pressure you've carried for years

Your body doesn't forget. It keeps score. It takes notes. And eventually… it asks to be heard. We store more than trauma. We store success, too — when it came at a cost. We store pressure. Expectations. The effort it took to *hold it all together* while smiling.

Tension is unspoken truth. Fatigue is your nervous system waving the white flag. And chronic pain is often your body saying, *"You've been carrying this too long."*

This isn't weakness. It's *wisdom*.

Because the body isn't betraying you. It's trying to bring you back.

When You Push Through — and Your Body Pushes Back

You can push through for a while. A long while, actually. You can keep smiling, keep producing, keep showing up. Even while exhausted. Even while aching. Even while quietly falling apart.

Until one day — your body says: *enough*.
It might start subtly:

- A recurring pain that no one can quite diagnose
- That low-level fatigue that sleep doesn't fix
- A tight chest when your phone buzzes
- The headaches, the tension, the digestive issues, the back pain — all the ways your body starts whispering

And then? If you don't listen, it stops whispering. It shouts. At first you think, *"This is inconvenient."* But it's not a disruption. It's a message. Your body isn't betraying you. It's protecting you — from the pace, the pressure, the pattern.

It's not failure.

It's a boundary.

And if you can stop seeing the crash as the end — and start seeing it as your body finally advocating for you — something beautiful starts to shift.

Breakdown Isn't Failure — It's Feedback

We're taught to see breakdown as the end. A collapse. A crisis. A problem to fix as fast as possible. But what if it's not failure? What if it's feedback? What if the crash is your body's clearest message — a redirection toward what's real, sustainable, and actually healing?

We push until something breaks. And then we say, *"What's wrong with me?"*

But maybe nothing's wrong. Maybe something's finally right — because now, at last, you're listening. The breakdown doesn't mean you're weak. It means you've been strong for too long — without rest, without help, without pause. It's the point at which the body stops negotiating.

And here's the thing. Sometimes the most powerful thing you can do... is fall apart *on purpose.*

Rest. Stop. Rethink. Heal.

This isn't giving up. It's a reset. The message is not "you can't go on."

It's "you shouldn't keep going like *that.*"

Reconnecting Without Fear

After burnout, illness, trauma, or even years of over-functioning, coming back into your body can feel... strange. You might feel numb. Or twitchy. Or just *tired of feeling* altogether. There's often a quiet fear:

If I really slow down and listen... what will I find?

And that fear makes sense.

Because the body remembers.

But here's the other truth. The body *also* remembers how to heal. It holds your resilience. Your wisdom. Your softness. Your calm. Reconnection doesn't have to be dramatic.

It starts with small invitations:

- Sitting still for two minutes — without reaching for your phone
- Moving in a way that feels good, not punishing
- Breathing into the parts that feel tight
- Noticing where you feel something — and not rushing to fix it

You don't have to dive back in. You don't have to force presence. You just have to start *being with yourself* again — gently, with curiosity instead of control.

And over time...the fear gives way to trust.

Listening Differently Now

Once you start listening, your body speaks. It won't shout. It won't send calendar invites. But it will nudge. Whisper. Tighten. Soften. Signal.

You begin to notice things you used to ignore:

- The shallow breath when something feels off
- The tension in your shoulders before you say "yes" to something you don't want to do
- The tiredness that no amount of sleep touches
- The lump in your throat when you're holding back truth
- The heaviness that follows a certain room, person, or conversation

This is your body's language. And it's honest — always. This isn't about becoming hyper-aware of every ache or flutter. It's about building trust. Pattern recognition. Response.

You stop asking, *"Am I being too sensitive?"* And start asking, *"What is this telling me?"* You don't need to outsource your truth. It's already in your system.

The more you listen, the clearer it becomes. And soon, your body stops being something you drag through life — and becomes something you lead *with*.

* * *

One day, I realised I wasn't tired. After chemo. After radiotherapy. After sleepless nights and deep, bone-level exhaustion. After stress that lived in my muscles and settled behind my eyes.

I was sitting quietly. Nothing dramatic. And it landed softly in me: *I'm not tired.* Just for that moment, I felt it. Clear. Present. Awake.

Not wired. Not pushing through. Just... *well.*

It felt like being reunited with a version of myself I hadn't seen in years. It didn't shout. It didn't announce itself with banners. But it was there.

* * *

The Archive in Your Bones

Your body is more than a machine. It's an archive. Not chaotic or random — but organised, layered, precise. A quiet library that holds your life in the fibres of your muscles, the rhythm of your breath, the tension in your jaw. It remembers the weight you carried — even when you smiled. The words you didn't say — even when you performed calm. The joy you felt before you were taught to tone it down. The grief that never quite had space to land.

Every ache, every sigh, every flutter of adrenaline — it's all data. A record. A trace.

The good news? You can update the archive. You can breathe into old tension and soften it. You can stretch into spaces that once held fear — and feel free. You can rewrite the patterns by *moving differently, choosing differently, listening differently*.

You're not stuck with the old story. Your body is holding it because it was never safe to let it go.

But now?

You're safe enough to release it. And when you do... you don't lose yourself.

You come home to yourself.

Reflection — What Is Your Body Trying to Tell You?

This isn't about analysing every ache. It's about noticing — with kindness. Your body has been keeping score. Not to punish you, but to communicate with you. Every tension. Every tight breath. Every restless night. It's all data.

It's all whispering something your mind might have been too busy — or too afraid — to hear. What if your body wasn't something to fight... but something to *trust*?

Journal Moment

- Where do you feel tension first when life gets overwhelming — your jaw, shoulders, stomach, chest?
- What parts of your body have been quietly carrying the cost of your pace or pressure?
- When did you last feel fully present in your body — safe, grounded, strong, or still?
- What has your body been trying to say... that your mind has been overriding?
- What might shift if you listened more and forced less?

You don't have to fix everything. You don't have to heal it all today. You just have to begin the conversation — and believe your body when it speaks. Because your body isn't a burden. It's not broken.

It's your oldest witness. And your wisest ally.

Pause. Reflect. Realign.

Your body remembers what your mind forgets.
 It's not here to slow you down — it's here to guide you home.
 Let it speak.

Let it lead.
Let it be the truth-teller you've been looking for.

Edge Move — Honour the Signal

This week, honour one signal your body gives you.

- Say no when your stomach flips.
- Rest before you hit the wall.
- Stretch, walk, sleep, breathe — without justifying it.
- Let a tear fall instead of blinking it back.
- Choose silence when your chest says *not now*.

You don't need to ask permission to feel. Just listen. And respond. Your body remembers. And now — it's ready to be met with respect.

Epilogue

This Is Not the End — Just a Deeper Beginning

If you've made it to this page, you already know. This wasn't a book about becoming *more*. It was about remembering who you already are — without the noise, without the mask, without the rush.

The journey wasn't linear. It wasn't polished. It was layered, textured, quiet, real. And that's how life is, too. You don't need to do more. You don't need to be louder, faster, or clearer than you are right now. You just need to keep choosing alignment over performance.

Wholeness over perfection.

Presence over pressure.

You've done that simply by being here. If something in you softened while reading — hold on to that. If something shifted — honour it. If something still feels uncertain — good. That's how real change begins.

This is not the end.

Andrea Ubhi

Just a deeper beginning.

Thank you for walking to the edge with me — and for having the courage to stay there long enough to see what might grow.

Lead gently. Stand fully. Live wide and quiet and true.

You've already arrived.

Afterword

The Heart Behind the Words

If this book stirred something in you — even just a flicker of courage or clarity — I'd love to tell you about the heartbeat behind it all.

> **100% of proceeds from this book go to Asha Nepal — and over 10% of annual profits from Andrea Ubhi Dentistry do too.**

This isn't a side project. This is central to who I am, and how I show up in the world.

Asha Nepal is a grassroots organisation supporting women and children who've survived trafficking, abuse, and exploitation. I have the privilege of serving as Chair — and the even greater privilege of walking alongside some of the bravest people I've ever met.

Asha means *hope*.

And hope is exactly what we help rebuild — not through

Afterword

rescue alone, but through education, long-term care, safe homes, deep community, and the quiet power of being believed in.

These women and girls are my greatest teachers. They are why I lead. Why I speak up. Why I keep showing up. Their resilience shapes the way I live — and everything I write.

Thank you for being part of something bigger. For believing in strength that doesn't shout. And for holding space for hope — in all its quiet, radical forms.

If you'd like to support, witness, or share in this work:
www.asha-nepal.org

Let's Stay in Touch

This might be the last page... but it doesn't have to be the last conversation. If this book met you somewhere real, I'd love to hear from you.

You can find me, my writing, and all the quiet adventures to come right here:

www.andreaubhi.com/edge

Afterword

And if this book supported you — helped you breathe a little deeper or feel a little more seen — a short review means the world. Your words help this reach the people who need it most.

Thank you for reading. For feeling. For walking the edge.

With love,
    Andrea x

Acknowledgments

This book began at the edge.

Not with a perfect plan or polished outline — but with truth breaking through the noise.

To everyone who's held space for my becoming —thank you. You may not know the part you played, but your presence, your questions, your listening, helped shape these pages.

To my children — you've been my greatest mirrors and my fiercest joy. Thank you for letting me evolve in front of you.

To the women and girls of Asha Nepal — your strength, your light, your fierce resilience have shaped my understanding of what true courage looks like. You are the heart of so much of this work. It is an honour to stand beside you.

To the women who offered their stories for this book — thank you for your courage and generosity. Your honesty threads through these pages like gold. You reminded me — and every reader — that strength takes many forms, and none of them need to shout.

To the women I've written this for — and to the women who have shaped me — thank you for your soft strength, your honesty, and your refusal to settle for a life that no longer fits. You helped me find my voice again. And now, I hope this helps you find yours.

To the team at Andrea Ubhi Dentistry — thank you for your brilliance, humour, and heart. You've made space for me to explore the mountain — and return, again and again, better for it.

And finally — to the version of me who couldn't see this far ahead, but kept walking anyway — thank you. You made it.

About the Author

Dr. Andrea Ubhi is an award-winning entrepreneur, adventurer, and advocate for calm, courageous living. As founder of Andrea Ubhi Dentistry and Chair of the charity Asha Nepal, Andrea has spent three decades leading from the front — until life invited her to lead from the edge instead.

After navigating burnout, serious illness, and a profound personal shift, she began rethinking everything: ambition, identity, success.

Lead from the Edge is the book she wished she'd had during that time — a guide for anyone ready to stop performing and start becoming.

Andrea lives between the Lake District and Yorkshire, and spends her time working, writing, climbing mountains, mentoring, and allowing music to find her feet in unexpected places — all with equal presence and purpose.

Connect to Andrea's world: www.andreaubhi.com/edge

Printed in Dunstable, United Kingdom